Sex Position for Couples

From Kama Sutra to Tantric Sex, Sex Games and Dirty Talks

TABLE OF CONTENTS

Copyright © 2019
COPYRIGHT PROTECTION

INTRODUCTION

We realize that the more inventive and the greater sexual repertoire we have, the more prominent the possibility of keeping up a good sex life. If I served you up a similar dinner, simultaneously of day, in a similar seat, at a similar table, you would before long get exhausted and uninterested. We have to recall that sexual activity is a lot of the equivalent; we need variety, that thrill of trying something new together. It is this that keeps us as intrigued by sex as it does in eating.

Unfortunately, a few couples become acclimated to engaging in sexual relations at a specific time of day, with the lights off, three minutes of foreplay and afterward intercourse. At the point when we experience the various phases of our life, we regularly need to adjust to family and work conditions. It isn't remarkable, for example, for a recently hitched couple to organize their affection making, since it is new and energizing, at that point kids go along. Even though the couple might want to have customary sexual action, the lady may think, "I would be wise to get this over rapidly if the youngsters wake up", or, when the kids are more established they think "I would be advised to be mindful so as not to make an excessive amount of clamor in case they comprehend what we are up to".

Parents regularly feel that it would be so humiliating if their kids knew that they are having intercourse. We react to this by having quick sex, and albeit a 'fast in and out' can be fun in the correct conditions, it is so natural to get into an unfortunate propensity and disregard the intimacy of sex, having the opportunity to snuggle and talk and explore one another's bodies as opposed to simply going for orgasm.

The principle issue with having such a small repertoire of sexual activity and not evaluating various methods for pleasuring each other, or distinctive sexual positions, is this: when we get older, and our bodies are experiencing joint inflammation, back agony, or we have had ongoing medical procedure, for example, a hip substitution or significant heart medical procedure, we will regularly need to change or adjust our sexual positions, so we don't feel torment or get cramp, or to evade the stress that we may harm ourselves some way.

If we have never discussed various types of intimate contact and have not discussed our sexual experiences, at that point if we get sick, it is quite a lot harder to change. I think this is mostly because when a partner is sick, one of the couples turns into a carer for some time, and this adjusts the dynamic in the relationship. Carers shouldn't ask for their needs to be met and so intimacy is often put to one side. A year or two later, couples state, "Everything began when my wife had a hip substitution and began sleeping downstairs", or "When my husband had prostate issues, I would not like to inconvenience him. Since he is better I couldn't want anything more than to have him back in bed with me; however, we have used to this new sleep schedule".

CHAPTER ONE

SEX POSITION FOR COUPLES

The missionary is the most commonly adopted lovemaking position since it is so comfortable. Yet, there are various methods of enjoying each other's bodies, and every one of the positions written on the next page may propose another into which you can move.

More intimacy is offered by certain situations' with all-over body contact and the chance to grasp and kiss, others offer further infiltration, some are very hard to keep up, which makes a specific desire to move urgency and excitement.

Adventurous lovers will discover varieties of their own, either by structure or by some coincidence: you may get overwhelmed by desire most of the way up the stairs or while talking in the kitchen. The significant thing is to connect every one of your instincts and feelings while remaining intensely mindful of your partner's responses.

Below are AWESOME sex positions to try:

Astride

With the man lying on his back on the bed, the lady can sit straddling him and control the pace of their lovemaking. Confronting him, she may squat on her hindquarters for an all the more dominant bobbing development, or, as here, stoop, supporting herself with her hands. Along these lines, she is allowed to lean forward and kiss his mouth. From this position, it is simple for her to build the closeness by lying with her entire body along with his. A variety is for her to confront away from him, expanding the profundity of infiltration.

Creep

Profound infiltration can be accomplished with the lady on every one of the fours and her accomplice bowing behind her. This position offers the two sweethearts the chance to push against each other, and the man may likewise touch his accomplice's bosoms, hindquarters, and clitoris. Back passage positions like this one are perfect when the two accomplices are in the disposition for lively as opposed to delicate lovemaking. A variety is for the two accomplices to remain with the lady bowing forward and supporting herself against furniture.

Cross

Here the lady lies on her back on the bed, and the man lies corner to corner over her. She opens her legs to enable him to enter and he shakes tenderly from side to side. She can direct his developments with the weight of her hands. This position is to some degree simpler to keep up if the man lies underneath on his back and the lady is in charge.

Cuissade

This position is known as 'cuissade', from the French cuisse, meaning thigh. The lady lies on her back, with the man next to her. She raises the leg closest to him and lays it on his body, and he enters from under her thigh, with his closest leg crossing her body. They can hold each other and kiss, and the position is an extremely private one, perhaps as a result of the 'cryptic' type of passage. The lady can apply a specific measure of limitation with her thigh, which can make it all the more energizing.

Cunnilingus

In cunnilingus, the man animates his accomplice's vulva and clitoris with his lips and tongue. For most ladies, cunnilingus gives the most flavorful exotic delight and is the ideal method for peaking. It is additionally incredibly exciting for her accomplice.

Cunnilingus - Oral sex upon a vulva

What is cunnilingus?

Cunnilingus is the compelling artwork of having intercourse with a vagina with your mouth and tongue. It is sensitive expertise, requiring tolerance, practice, and commitment to take care of business, yet any lady you figure out how to do it directly for will welcome all of you the more for it.

What applies to the penis applies to the vulva-everybody is unique, requiring an alternate touch to fulfill its proprietor. Yet, not many instruments can rise to the tongue for the measure of delight it can convey to a glad vagina.

This segment expects that you recognize what a vulva resembles and can relate to some accuracy the mons veneris, labia majora, clitoral hood, clitoris, labia minora, urethra, vagina, and perineum, to name them (roughly) start to finish.

How quick would it be a good idea for me to go?

This isn't an assault. Try not to pursue the clitoris like a firefighter assaulting a fire. Regularly from the start, the clitoris is unreasonably touchy for direct incitement. Lick around it, invigorating the hood, prodding her internal labia, tasting her. Take as much time as is needed and hear her out. A few ladies make a clamor, and some don't. It will be some time before you realize precisely what your sweetheart lean towards to the extent oral sex is concerned. A few ladies may like extra incitement - a finger or two into the vagina, or maybe even the rear-end. She may need your hands to reach up and play with her bosoms, or she may need your fingers to hold her labia separated so your tongue can get at her vulva all the more straightforwardly.

I've heard cunnilingus doesn't taste great

If the taste or smell irritates you or is a worry, request that her wash first. A great many people who appreciate cunnilingus concur that a perfect vagina is a decent, whenever obtained, taste. As a lady approaches her peak, she may need more straightforward incitement. When all is said in done, quick, cadenced incitement is best at causing peak - yet there shouldn't be a race to arrive. Take as much time as necessary and figure out how to acknowledge what you can accomplish for her.

Shouldn't something be said about cunnilingus during a monthly cycle?

A few people are especially skilled at the recommendation of cunnilingus during the feminine cycle. If it is a worry to you, at that point pause, a tampon may well keep the blood down, as will a stomach, yet a few men can't stand the taste in any case. If your accomplice is solid, in any case, there is no specific threat in menstrual blood, and a few ladies find that climaxes during their period's alleviated cramps.

Fellatio

In fellatio, the lady sucks licks, kisses, and strokes her accomplice's penis. Flawlessly fulfilling for the man, fellatio can likewise give huge sensual joy to the lady as she detects his reactions and his complete relinquishment to her.

Fellatio - Oral sex upon a penis
What is Fellatio?

Fellatio, giving head, giving a sensual caress, numerous men love this sort of incitement, and numerous individuals, the two ladies, and men, such as giving it. Fellatio is the demonstration of applying your lips to a man's penis to give him delight.

There are scarcely any tips to fellatio that can be given other than training. The lips and the tongue are the significant wellsprings of incitement, and it is with the lips and tongue that you ought to apply the consideration regarding make him feel better. The two people react well to weight and cadence. A relentless, solid stroke will be sufficient to get the response you're searching for.

Imagine a scenario in which it doesn't smell or taste pleasant.

If the smell isn't something you appreciate, at that point guide him to go wash up! While this is something you're doing principally for his pleasure, that doesn't mean you need to endure if he's inadequate in cleanliness! What's more, in case you're stressed over germs, your mouth has millions a greater number of germs than a perfect penis.

What is "profound throating?"

Profound throating is the demonstration of bringing the penis down past your muffle reflex. In all actuality, this specific sexual experience is very misrepresented. The ideal approach to give fellatio is still with the lips and tongue, accepting just as much as you can without choking. Nonetheless, for those that need to know, the fundamental exercise is still practice. Accept the penis to the extent you can without gagging, and afterward, close your eyes and concentrate, taking each quarter-inch, revealing to yourself that you won't gag, that you can take it out whenever, and gradually swallow it down. At that point, ascend off of it similarly as gradually.

Are there any extraordinary spots on the penis?

Each penis is unique, and every one has its soft spots and its favored methods for being taken care of. Tune in to your sweetheart. The sounds he makes and the vibe of his body straining are your best hints that you're going this right.

Would it be advisable for me to utilize my hands?

Don't hesitate to get a handle on with your hands whatever of the penis you can't fit into your mouth. Numerous men like however much incitement as could reasonably be expected and the vibe of a wet mouth and a spit slicked hand are sufficient to send them to the edge of climax rapidly.

What are 69?

A few people feel that the best position to perform oral sex is the 69 position, where each accomplice lies with their head by the other's privates. For fellatio, this even bodes well - most penises bend upwards, towards the head, and in this position bend coordinates the bend of the throat. Be that as it may, it is hard to both perform and acknowledge oral sex simultaneously. Attempt the position, or bow by his body, however at any rate before all else does each thing in turn.

My beau needs me to swallow. What do I do?

Which carries us to a touchy issue: gulping discharge, for some men, this is critical to them- - they like to feel that by gulping their semen, you complete this demonstration of lovemaking and acknowledge a piece of themselves into your body. Be that as it may, numerous individuals don't care for the flavor of semen and can't bring themselves. Discussion about this in advance let him know whether you can't deal with it and that it's not close to home.

Would I be able to make my seminal fluids taste better?

Macrobiotic nutritionists have done research on this inquiry, and the appropriate response is in: the type of food you eat will affect your general health. The presence of mind directs that if you taste great, your sweetheart will need to eat you all the more regularly, so improving your body's taste and smell ought to be imperative to you. As a rule, nutritionists state that antacid based nourishments, for example, meets and fish produce margarine, fish taste.

Dairy items, which contain a high bacterial festering level, make the foulest tasting liquids by a wide margin. (Difference: nearly everybody I know says that there is one more terrible than high-dairy content- - asparagus. You can't miss the flavor of asparagus-bound semen.) Acidic natural products, for example, desserts, organic products, and liquor give natural liquids a wonderful, sugary flavor. Synthetically prepared mixers will cause a very acidic taste, be that as it may, so in case you're going to drink liquor, drink high-caliber, normally aged lagers (Rolling Rock or Kirin) or purpose.

What are the substances of semen?

The subject of semen content emerges particularly among people who routinely swallow semen, as in fellatio, and who are worried about calorie consumption and nourishing substances. The normal discharge contains aboutonia, ascorbic corrosive, blood-bunch antigens, calcium, chlorine, cholesterol, choline, citrus extract, creatine, deoxyribonucleic corrosive (DNA), fructose, glutathione, hyaluronidase, inositol, lactic corrosive, magnesium, nitrogen, phosphorus, potassium, purine, pyrimidine, pyruvic corrosive, sodium, sorbitol, spermidine, spermine, urea, uric corrosive, nutrient b12, and zinc.

The caloric substance of a normal discharge is assessed to be around 15 calories. There is just one genuine approach to do fellatio, and that is with excitement. You need to cherish what you're doing to him, either because you love him or you love sucking cockerel. Cherishing both is ideal! Faked climaxes have nothing on dull fellatio.

Fireside

In this comfortable position, which can pursue cunnilingus, the lady sits easily in a rocker with her hands and legs around the man, who enters bowing before her. On the off chance that she reclines, he can bolster himself with his hands on the rear of the seat, which will permit him more push.

Futon

For this position, you have to evaluate all your furniture to discover a bit of the right tallness. The lady lies on the edge of a table, futon or bed secured with blankets and cushions, and spreads her legs wide. The man can start by bowing to give her cunnilingus, at that point he enters her, supporting himself on his knees and holding her legs. This bears him a lot of control, and the edge of infiltration is steep.

Head to toe

The man lies on his back with his legs spread and his penis inside the lady, who additionally rests on her back, with her legs spread over his, her toes indicating his head, and her head away from him. The lady is in charge. The accomplices can't see one another and sensation is focused on the private parts. This position can be embraced from one in which the sweethearts sit on the bed confronting each other, their legs intertwined.

Lap

This is a place that may present itself while nestling on the couch. The man sits with the lady straddling his lap, confronting him. She controls the pace, they can kiss, and he can stroke her bosoms. She goes here and there on him, supporting herself with her knees on the couch, and her arms around his neck. On the off chance that they utilize an eating seat, she can keep her feet on the floor and clutch the seat back for help if fundamental. If she faces from him, they will have the option to accomplish further entrance, and she could bolster herself against furniture before her.

Missionary

The Missionary position is the most well-known lovemaking position of all since it is agreeable, manages a lot of body contact and great profundity of infiltration. The darlings can kiss and hold each other simultaneously. The lady lies on her back with her legs spread and her knees raised, and her accomplice lies on top between her legs. From this position, the lady can move to fasten her legs despite her accomplice's good faith or to close them firmly underneath him, while he spreads his.

CHAPTER TWO

SEX IN PREGNANCY

Except if your primary care physician reveals to you else, it is consummately alright for you to engage in sexual relations all through your pregnancy. Be that as it may, towards the normal birth date, your size may make numerous positions awkward for you. Infiltration might be least demanding if you lie on your side and your accomplice enters from behind. Oral sex and shared masturbation should cause no issues. A few ladies dread that sexual movement or climax may trigger off work yet sex can't prompt work except if the infant is expected in any case, when the prostaglandin present in the man's semen may make it start.

The sex drive of certain ladies diminishes during the primary trimester of pregnancy. This might be because of tiredness and sickness, or to a shrouded conviction that it isn't 'right' for a mother to appreciate sex. The issue will, for the most part, vanish voluntarily. In certain ladies, the sex drives increments during the center three months (the subsequent trimester) of pregnancy, and in some cases that their lovemaking is more fulfilling than any other time in recent memory. This might be because the elevated level of flowing hormones implies that a lady can be animated all the more effectively and arrive at a pitch of sexual fervor more rapidly than when not pregnant. A pregnant lady's sexual organs bosoms, areolas, and private parts - are particularly exceptionally created, which presumably increments sexual mindfulness. At last, there is finished opportunity from the stress of getting pregnant, which permits a more profound degree of 'giving up'.

A few ladies and their accomplices stress that sex may hurt the unborn youngster, yet such apprehensions are baseless. The baby is shielded from disease by the attachment of bodily fluid at the neck of the belly. In uncommon cases, contamination can occur; however, this is for the most part because of the absence of typical cleanliness safety measures or engaging in sexual relations with a few unique accomplices. The infant is additionally ensured against being squashed by the amniotic liquid in which it glides in the belly. Keep away from over-athletic sex since it will be awkward for you, yet don't stress over harming the child. Sex ought not to cause premature delivery in a typical, sound pregnancy.

You can continue sex after labor when it is agreeable to do as such, ladies who have had an episiotomy (in which the perineum is sliced to encourage birth), will presumably feel sore for at any rate three weeks. At the point when you feel certain that your injury has recuperated, start to restore your sexual coexistence, taking it gradually and delicately and utilizing a greasing up jam if important to anticipate scar tissue causing uneasiness or torment. It is essential to build up sexual contact with your accomplice when you can, as you will both need to draw near once more. On the off chance that regardless you feel sore, recollect there are different methods for giving and getting friendship. Try not to let your accomplice feel that you are showering all your consideration and consideration on your child and barring him from your affection.

Positions for pregnancy

Spoons

The lady lies serenely on her side, and the man enters her from behind, accommodating his body near hers. This position puts no weight on the lady's midriff and is reasonable for the most developed phases of pregnancy. The man can nestle very close and stroke her bosoms while kissing her shoulders and the scruff of her neck.

Leapfrog

The lady bows on the bed with legs spread wide and falls easily advances as the man enters her from behind. He would then be able to touch her back and control the profundity of push. This position is perfect when the lady begins to feel awkward with the man's weight pushing down on her, and she needs to shield her midsection from over-energetic pushing.

Astride

This is a decent position for the center a very long time of pregnancy when the teacher position has gotten awkward; however, the lady has a lot of vitality for sex. She sits on the back of the man's lap and supports herself with her arms. He can help her as she goes all over him, taking control when she gets worn out.

CHAPTER THREE

SENSUOUS SEDUCTION

The blinds are shut, the candlelight is gleaming, the beverages are cooling. All you need presently are some smooth moves to lure your darling endlessly from the rigors of the day and into your softening grasp. Continuously remember that no temptation is finished without some genuine kissing, Kama Sutra-style. In any case, the old writings demand that, when you've stimulated your darling with a kiss, you should be set up to catch up with other enchanting aptitudes.

The accompanying pages tell you the best way to entice in style. Pick your system and apply it with all the alluring authority you can gather. On the off chance that you decide to strip your sweetheart, strip off the layers such that fringes on respectful. If you decide on an exotic grasp, make it time-halting serious. If you treat your accomplice to some oral cherishing, give them that there's no spot on the planet you'd preferably be. Whatever you do, commit yourself, brain and body, to the occasion.

Enchantment

Enchantment can occur in the wink of an eye or the sending of an underhandedly express instant message. It can likewise be a lengthier, waiting issue, in which you can utilize the procedures appeared here. In any case, take your lead from the Kama Sutra and make temptation your top need.

The must-have-it state of mind

It's anything but difficult to jump on your sweetheart when you're in the temperament. The test comes when they're NOT in the mind-set. Perhaps they've quite recently gotten back home from work; possibly they have stuff at the forefront of their thoughts. Your responsibility is to transform them around and get them into an absolute necessity have-it disposition.

What's more, to do this, you need some hot enticement methods added to your repertoire. Attempt any of the accompanying to drive your darling wild with want: Call your sweetheart when you're only minutes from meeting them. Stimulate their feeling of expectation by disclosing to them that you're horny to the point that you need to engage in sexual relations straight away. Instruct them to get ready in like manner. Or then again, on the off chance that you need to speak to your darling's feeling of fun, have a go at luring them with sheer fun-loving nature. Challenge them to a pad battle or spruce up in their clothing and request that they strip you.

Reverse the situation

In case you're generally the one to tempt and start in your sexual coexistence, take a stab at shaking things up with some invert brain research. Tell your accomplice that you're going on a sex "detox" for a couple of days, the clue that you could be convinced to break your quick if the correct sort of allurement tagged along. You'll see a different side of them as they battle to get you into bed.

The intensity of the psyche

On the off chance that you can fill your darling's head with desire and lustfulness, you may find that their body is chomping at the bit to go before you even touch them. Take a stab at requesting that your darling depicts in detail a provocative demonstration they'd prefer to perform on you.

Sensual proposal

Pursue Vatsyayana's recommendation and enjoy some hot visit to get things moving: "… talk intriguingly of things that would be viewed as coarse, or not to be referenced in the public eye."

Playing with artfulness

Show your provocative aims by improving the bed with blossom petals. At that point, drag your accomplice into the room for some classic being a tease and caressing, so they know precisely what you have as a top priority.

Setting the mind-set

You can likewise set the disposition dial to tempting by accomplishing something exciting together, for example, slow and attractive moving. Start dressed and help each other gradually strip as the move warms up.

Grasps

A sensual grasp can take the sexual state of mind from lukewarm to torrid in the flutter of an eyelash. Little contrasts to the experience of standing and your body in a tight secure against your lover's. It enables you to put every one of the burdens and strains of the world behind you and to enter the domain of your faculties.

Outside satisfactions

The antiquated sensual writings are joined regarding the matter of grasps: they are fundamental primers to the demonstration of adoration. The Ananga Ranga alludes to them as "outside delights" that "ought to consistently go before interior satisfactions." Their main responsibility is to "build up the craving... These influence and redirect the psyche from bashfulness and frigidity." Embraces are imperative to the point that they are recorded for each event, a portion of the grasps that the Kama Sutra suggests, for example, The Twining of a Creeper, ought to be "performed at the hour of welcome a sweetheart," and are expected as sexy articulations of friendship. Others, for example, The Embrace of Milk and Water, are proposed to get you boiling with anger.

Receiving the benefits

The message is truly basic: invest bunches of energy grasping in the development of sex. Embraces, strokes, snog, and nestles increase the sexual pressure, so sex turns out to be progressively dangerous when you get down to it. What's more, don't spare grasps only for sex; make them part of regular daily existence with the goal that any minute can be erotic. Embrace hi, lie weaved while you're viewing a film, and bid farewell with a hot full-body grasp.

The puncturing grasp

She squeezes her bosoms against his body in an energetic I-need you right-now signal he won't have the option to stand up to. He cups her bosoms in his grasp and strokes them delicately.

The twining of the creeper

She sticks to his body with every one of her appendages "as a creeper twines cycle a tree." She twists his head towards her face so she can look at him affectionately before kissing him delicately and exotically.

The grasp of milk and water

She sits on his lap and wraps herself firmly around him. He holds her nearby in his arms. The way that your privates are in such closeness is a genuine turn-on. Envision that is no joke "go into one another's bodies."

The squeezing grasp

Defeat by desire, he squeezes her against a divider and moves in to cover her body with his. Take a stab at pounding your hips together to get the sexual strain moving; you presumably won't have the option to control yourselves.

CHAPTER FOUR

ORAL SEX

Oral sex starts with the main profound kiss, and proceeds with kisses everywhere throughout the body, focusing at last on the private parts. Concerning the supplier, it requires a level of the enthusiastic association since it must be finished with persistence, delicacy, affectability, and mounting; however, controlled energy if it is to be great. Sweethearts who give oral sex hesitantly and without liberality or delight make their accomplices feel regretful and narrow-minded, and excessively tense and stressed to unwind and take joy themselves.

Inappropriate, against the ethical code, and not for courteous learned fellows was the Kama Sutra's assessment of oral sex. However, that didn't prevent Vatsyayana from depicting in delicious detail precisely how a eunuch or male hireling should bow between his lord's legs and "suck the mango" or "gobble up".

From the recipient, oral sex requires trust and the certainty that accompanies being made to feel attractive. In sex, as indifferent everyday issues, it is frequently more hard to get liberality than to give it; however, the individual who surrenders totally to joy conveys oneself over to the darling, and this additionally gives a feeling of wonderment. It's a given that sexual cleanliness is of prime significance for any individual who takes part in oral sex.

Oral sex for ladies is called cunnilingus. For some ladies, cunnilingus is the most energizing of the considerable number of varieties of sex, and a delicate and skillful darling ought to have the option to make his accomplice accompany his tongue more effectively than in some other manner. A solid tricky tongue can be utilized with exactness on the clitoris without risk of causing any torment, in contrast to a finger.

Start by kissing your accomplice's face and mouth, and afterward, bit by bit work your way down her body, kissing and stroking her bosoms, tummy, and internal thighs. Flick your tongue in light, fluffy kisses along the plump creases of the external labia, smoothing the pubic hair endlessly and afterward separating the labia tenderly with your fingers. Move slowly inwards with your tongue. Differ your developments as per your accomplice's reaction. Have a go at nestling, tunneling, pushing with your tongue into her vagina, sucking, long sensitive licks, and short quick flicking licks. She dislikes her clitoris to be animated straightforwardly from the outset, so continue probably until she is completely stirred.

When she can confide in YOU and feel sure that you like what you are doing, she will be capable completely to give up in the climax. Being 'on the detect', a man can get a unique rush from encountering so straightforwardly the euphoric impact he has on his accomplice, just as from her helplessness and trust.

Oral sex for men is called fellatio. The experience of having their penis sucked, licked and kissed is one that most men find strongly energizing. Now and again, there might be mental obstructions to survive. A few men dread being chomped during oral sex. The lady should open her mouth as wide as could be allowed, and close her lips, yet not her teeth, over the penis. Utilizing every one of the muscles in the lips and tongue will imply that the teeth should not come into contact with the penis by any means.

A few ladies are concerned that they might be stifled during fellatio. The best approach to alleviate this dread is to stay in charge: you are the person who should move while your accomplice lies still, so there is no plausibility of his pushing profound into your throat and making you choke. A few ladies consider gulping semen offensive. There is no requirement for you to do this on the off chance that you don't wish to, yet numerous ladies do appreciate having their accomplice discharge into their mouths.

Work your way down your accomplice's body, starting with kissing his face and mouth and advancing to his privates. Be delicate, as they are profoundly touchy to torment. There are numerous methods for invigorating the penis with your lips and tongue. You can lick up and down the pole with a sensitive tongue, at that point utilize more weight and press your open lips just as your tongue against it as you rub them all over towards the head. You can lick and kiss the frenulum - the delicate spot where the glans joins the pole on the underside, which will look towards you if the man is lying on his back with an erection. You can take the leader of the penis in your mouth and suck it, stimulating it simultaneously with your tongue, and you can move your lips as far down the pole as is agreeable. At that point go here and there, sucking and squeezing with your lips and tongue.

The '69' position is alleged because the figures take after a couple giving each other oral sex. While numerous couples locate this a decent method for stirring one another, others think that it is hard to focus on giving and accepting such exceptional joy simultaneously. On the off chance that you are going to come in this position, it is ideal to sever from pleasuring your accomplice to dodge unintentionally gnawing the person in question. Utilize your fingers to show to your accomplice what's going on and let yourself go in the climax.

Unsatisfactory practices
Fellatio in the Kama Sutra is absolutely a method for a worker to fulfill his lord in the middle of his loving undertakings. Vatsyayana favored not to recognize that a pure and delightful lady may go down on her if he mentions that "ladies of the group of concubines" may at times enjoy somewhat oral to breathe easy.

Oral sex to die for
If you do not have (or need) a helpful eunuch or group of concubines, you'll need to manage with one another. Albeit oral is an extraordinary method to warm each other up before sex, have a go at making it your principle course instead of only a starter. Realizing that your sweetheart is focused on going all the way is an amazing sexual enhancer. At the point when you're doing the giving, make it hot, wet, and wild. If your sweetheart sees that you're cherishing it, they'll love it much more. At the point when you're in a bad way, show your thankfulness as groans, moans, and "Mmmmm"s.

Regardless of anything else, take as much time as is needed. Bother before you go in for the kill. Linger on your sweetheart's inward thighs, perineum, or pubic triangle. Invest your energy kissing, tickling, nestling, and licking. Ensure that your sweetheart is humming with desire before you apply your lips to the clitoris or penis.

Intimate Union

The following sex positions are made for exotic sessions before a log fire, love-ins in a four-publication bed, or making out in a late spring glade or classic room. They are packed with sentiment, closeness, and soul-merging at the top of the priority list. Think tantric as opposed to torrid.

Here you can test the nose-to-nose adorableness of Butterflies in Flight, the radiantly close Singing Monkey, and the pleasures of the provocatively named Cat and Mouse Sharing a Hole. In any case, don't depend on the position alone to keep up that sentimental power; proceed with the seething eye to eye connection and fingertip strokes.

Similarly that you'd pick the correct wine to go with a delightful dinner, select the right sex strokes to go with the position, for example, profound pushing may work superbly in The Stopper-age, yet be awkward in Coitus from Behind. You can broaden your collection of sex strokes by adapting some old pushing procedures in The Movements of Sex.

Generally opened position

The lady has an unordinary measure of space to express her desire in this minor departure from the conventional man-on-top position. Since his hips are high noticeable all around instead of sticking her to the bed, she's allowed to push, granulate, and squirm as much as she needs.

Why it works

- You alternate to lead the pack: she pushes upward when it's her turn in control; he pushes descending when it's his.

- When she's the one making the moves, he encounters an exciting descending draw on his pole.
- You can tailor the situation to your state of mind. You can pummel your bodies against one another in wild forsake or make little, delicate developments in snapshots of heartfelt closeness.
- He doesn't put any weight on her, which is helpful if she's pregnant.

Two fishes and Swallows in affection

Attempt this pair of positions when you need prodding to develop to sex. The entrance is troublesome in Two Fishes so that you can go through it to slope the sexual pressure. At that point, when you're so tense you can't tolerate it any longer, she can move on to her back and open her legs wide in welcome.

Why they work
- Two Fishes is an extraordinary situation for bunches of skin-stroking, ass-grabbing, and profound kissing foreplay. It gives you both sufficient occasions to heat up and get your juices streaming.
- He can kick-start her excitement by slipping his hand around to stroke her labia and clitoris.
- Swallows in Love (a.k.a. the evangelist position) is a nitty-gritty man-on-top situation in which you're both allowed to focus on the in-out development of his penis.
- She can snatch his butt to impact the mood, pace, and profundity of his pushes, and rock her pelvis to his developments.

Parallel grasp

You both untruth straight and parallel on your sides, he envelops her with his arms as you kiss enthusiastically. He enables his hands to wander over her butt and thighs.

The snare

She shares her legs over the highest point of his in Two Fishes position. He pushes against her body without entering her.

Turning over

She turns over on to her back while he continues kissing her from the side.

Man on top He jumps over her, and she opens her legs to give him access. This is Swallows in Love. He takes his weight on his lower arms as he pushes unreservedly.

The principal act

This stance is suitably named because it's regularly the primary position that sweethearts get into when they need classic, man-on-top sex. It's not athletic, outlandish, or masterful, yet for basic, agreeable sweetness, it can't be beaten.

Why it works

- He gets the fulfillment of pushing openly and profoundly because her knees are raised.
- The shaft of his penis contacts her clitoris on each push, giving her significant erosion where she needs it most.
- You're very close, so the joy on your darling's face is plain to see. You can sustain off one another's excitement to drive the force of your lovemaking out of this world.
- Her hands are allowed to wander all over his body to make this position especially exotic just as sexual.

Midsection to stomach

Here and there, sex should be quick and upstanding. Perhaps you're doing it in the shower, or possibly you're outside and you can't rest. Whatever your setting, Belly to Belly is a most optimized plan of attack course to infiltration, without losing the closeness of vis-à-vis, skin-on-skin contact.

Why it works

- You can move on from kissing to out and out sex in a moment or two. The promptness of your desire is a love potion for both of you.
- You don't have to strip; she sneaks off her undies and lifts her skirt. He at that point drops his jeans, and away you go.
- His penis enters her at an irregular edge, making a lot of invigorating erosion against her clitoris and labia.
- You can make sex feel extra-filthy by disclosing to one another your naughtiest dreams, as you are at such lacking elbow room.

Catching and Side-by-side fastening

Catching is a hot variety of the preacher position in which she traps him with her feet around his legs. To blend things up mid-session, you turn over into a one next to the other position. What's more, if you need to, you can continue rolling with the goal that she has a turn on top as well.

Why they work

- If you both utilize a shaking movement in the Clasping position, she has a decent possibility of arriving at the climax. She shakes down while he shakes up.
- The Clasping position is probably the best position for nestling, embracing, snuggling, kissing, and kissing.
- Side-by-Side Clasping changes the rhythm and puts her on an increasingly equivalent premise; she can push to and fro while he stays still.
- Rolling on to your sides is a decent method to temper his desire and make sex last more if Clasping is pushing his catches too rapidly

Love's combination

This is what might be compared to a cup of cocoa: warm, supporting, and soothing. He takes her in his arms, and she cuddles against him as you tenderly rock against one another. What you pass up in confounding energy you'll compensate for in closeness, sentiment, and delicacy.

Why it works

- In this position, his penis bumps her vaginal passageway or infiltrates by only a modest quantity. This is beneficial for her because the external third of the vagina is the part that is generally delicate to incitement.
- He gets the opportunity to show his minding side by adopting a delicate and cherishing strategy to sex.
- There's no presentation pressure on her; she can lie back and feel snuggled and secure in his arms.
- Love's Fusion encourages you to bond when you've been away from one another, or to make up after you've had a contention.

Mandarin duck

This surprising position includes some requesting leg tangles; it may not be the quickest course to entrance and climax, yet it's amusing to attempt in case you're in an innovative, trial temperament. You can generally snicker and tumble your way into a simpler position on the off chance that it turns out badly

Why it works

- The point at which his penis enters her vagina may deliver some new and inebriating sensations.
- You both appreciate the fulfillment of giving something somewhat a shot of the customary.
- You can have a great time helping out one another to get into position.
- You'll be so engrossed with making sense of which leg ought to go where that you'll leave all your sexual restraints behind.
- You're vis-à-vis so that you can appreciate each other's demeanors of delight/diversion.

Squeezing and Twining

Praise your affection in these two sincerely charged positions. You're going to be secured an energetic vis-à-vis secure in which he does the squeezing, and she does the twining. So put the silk sheets on the bed, light the candles, and let the cherishing start.

Why they work

- Although he's in the predominant position, sex remains intuitive. She controls his energy by embracing his top half in her arms and encasing his base half between her legs.
- Pressing and Twining stream flawlessly into one another. There are a lot of other leg positions she can explore different avenues regarding as well, for example, moving her knee or fixing her leg.
- When he feels her heel on the rear of his leg in twining position, he realizes that she needs him more profound inside her.

- You can be as physically and genuinely close as you like in these positions; they're ideal for the can't-keep-your-hands-off one another phase of a relationship.

Butterflies in flight

Most well-known lady on-top positions highlight her sitting or bowing with on leg on each side of his abdomen and riding him cowgirl-style. A butterfly in Flight is increasingly delicate and alluring. She stays in control, while he gets the advantage of feeling all her erogenous zones moving tenderly down on his.

Why it works

- She can test and position herself with the goal that his penis enters her at the most suggestively fulfilling point.
- He encounters the energy of playing a latent job during sex. He's nailed somewhere around her body, and her hands and feet are over his, so it's hard for him to move.
- It's an opportunity to engage in sexual relations at a quieter pace than expected; you can both relish the unpretentious developments and sensations.
- She can propel herself all over in little however attractive developments with her arms, legs, and center quality, utilizing his feet as a stage.

Grasping with toes

The closeness of Gripping with Toes originates from his solid savage on-each of the fours stance encasing her helplessness. Since she's half suspended with her legs around his middle, she's for the most part subject to him to make the moves. Supporting this difficult situation for a whole sex session relies upon whether her thigh muscles can take care of business.

"Kisses, snack, sucking of lips, fastening of bosoms, and drinking energy-charged salivation are the things that make solid love. On the off chance that you do these things, the two discharges will happen all the while and pleasure will be finished for both of you."

Grasping with toes

Why it works

- If she has solid thigh muscles, she can give him tasty sensations by pulling herself all over on his body (consider pull-ups on an exercise center bar).
- He adores the sentiment of her legs bolted energetically around his middle.
- You can both experience the potent rush of oddity and the fulfillment of pulling off a dubious move; it is difficult to have intercourse when she's incompletely suspended.
- Her head is lower than her feet, so she gets a surge from being marginally reversed.
- Athletic positions, for example, this requires sexual collaboration. When you've taken a stab at Gripping with Toes, you'll need to push your sensual limits significantly further.

Transverse lute and Placid grasp

The mind-set is not tranquil in this smaller than expected grouping. After a serious kiss lying on your sides, you both turn over by 90 degrees with the goal that she's on her back. He at that point gets her and aides her onto his prepared and willing erection.

Why they work

- In the Placid Embrace, he can enter profoundly, and she can either watch the power of his longing or recline and appreciate the ride.
- Side-by-side positions, for example, the Transverse Lute imply that both of you can lead the pack in moving, kissing, and touching.
- The Transverse Lute additionally allows you to enjoy loads of spine-shivering foreplay and get under one another's skin before he enters.
- Moving from the Transverse Lute to the Placid Embrace makes an exciting state of mind change; she is cleared into his arms as he assumes responsibility.

The pine tree

This provocative position is alleged because the lady's raised legs take after the tall, exquisite trunk of a pine tree; ideal for tree-huggers all over the place. Attempt The Pine Tree when you're in the state of mind for sex that is X-appraised and hot, yet cherishing and close as well.

Why it works

- He's in a steady position that lets him control how quick and profound his developments are. Any varieties produce exciting sensations for both of you.
- Lying on her back with her legs extended straight noticeable all around makes her vibe supple and athletic, yet attractive as well.
- He gets a sensual frisson from being held under control by her legs as he enters her.
- She can fix him with a provocative look as he looks at her through her thighs.
- Her hands are allowed to delight both of you.

The fifth stance

This straightforward position is a great arousing blessing from him to her. His main responsibility is too luxurious her stripped body done with amazing touches while delicately having intercourse with her. Her activity is to lie back and appreciate: what more could any young lady request?

Why it works

- Because he doesn't infiltrate her completely, the delicate external third of her vagina gets a large portion of the consideration.
- She can concentrate only without anyone else joy with no strain to respond.
- He encounters the rush of making her dissolve.
- It's ideal for early morning wake-up sex; you're both warm and tired, and you get a delicate yet suggestive beginning to the day.

- If his erection travels every which way, it doesn't make a difference, because the accentuation is on erotic touch as opposed to immovable pushing.

The developments of sex

How you granulate your pelvis, go all over or undulate your entire body can affect unsurprising sex and unstable sex that will leave you limp and wheezing. Here are some development recommendations from the Kama Sutra and The Perfumed Garden.

On the off chance that you ordinarily siphon your approach to climax with no variety in style, pace, or beat, set yourself a test, imagine you've never had intercourse and need to make sense of how to move without any preparation. Attempt each sort of development from bobbing, shaking, scouring, and hovering to squirming, shaking, crawling, and undulating; and that implies both of you. Indeed, even take a stab at remaining still for the infrequent minute during sex. If you feel senseless, turn off the lights.

Stirring

This includes him taking the base of his pole immovably close by and whirling the tip of his penis along the length of her vulva. The primary feature of his visit ought to be her clitoris, utilizing to and fro flicks or firm circles, with periodic temporary re-routes to her vaginal passage, where he presses and beats his glans.

This can lead on to another prodding stroke known as Love's Tailor, in which he slips the tip of his penis a little route inside her and rubs it here and there. It is incredible for her because, as the Kama Sutra says, a "lady's tingle is generally broad in the external piece of her vagina." Then, exactly when she's becoming acclimated to shallow in-and-out developments, he can give her the rush of the unforeseen by all of the sudden diving in the whole distance. He can differ his strokes from shallow excessively profound all through sex.

Love's bond

This is the place he infiltrates her, so the full length of his penis is inside her, at that point delays for an ecstatic most extreme entrance minute. This can lead to the well-known in-and-out movement of intercourse; he can push more than once without pulling back, which is known as Sporting of a Sparrow. The Kama Sutra says this happens "toward the finish of intercourse." To make it as animating as could be expected under the circumstances, keep the developments light, liquid, and long. Another mid-sex method to attempt includes him pulling back totally and afterward reappearing at top speed, known as giving a Blow. It's not to everybody's taste; thus, on the off chance that you attempt it, pick an agreeable situation in which you can make certain of a smooth reemergence.

A lady putting on a show of a man

Every one of the strokes so far has been for men to do on ladies, yet the jobs can undoubtedly be turned around, so she is the dynamic party. The Kama Sutra likewise portrays how she can turn around on his penis in The Top, hold him firmly in The Mare, and rock on his penis in The Swing.

Rock with me

Sex specialists regularly prescribe a shaking procedure to assist ladies with arriving at the climax. She lies on her back with him on top. His careful position is significant: he needs to "enjoy some real success" on her body with the goal that the base of his penis is scouring toward her clitoris. He can accomplish this by infiltrating her, at that point shimmying up her body until he can't get any higher without his penis sneaking out. Presently you start the immensely significant shaking. As she shakes her pelvis down toward the bed, he shakes his toward the roof. This pulls a huge piece of his pole out of her. Next, she shakes her pelvis toward the roof as he shakes his toward the bed. This brings his whole penis back inside her, causing tight, sliding rubbing against her clitoris. Rehash until peak!

Singing monkey

She takes control in this agreeable yet provocative lady on-top position. It's sex at its slowest and sauciest. It's likewise an extraordinary open door for her to get him a sensual exhibition where she flaunts her body. He, in the interim, kicks back and appreciates the ride.

Why it works

- Her legs are spread wide, so entrance is profound and simple, and she can without much of a stretch animate her clitoris with her fingers.
- She can investigate various sensations by reclining on her hands to change the point at which his penis enters her.
- It's a sure and attractive situation wherein you can take as much time as is needed, recline on your hands, and value one another.
- You can kiss, however much you might want. Start with provisional lip and tongue contacts, and progress to an exceptional mouth-merging that flabbergasts you.

Cicada on a branch

He crawls up and takes her from behind in this smooth variation of sex. You both get all the unusual sensations and advantages of back section sex, but since you're not down on each of the fours, it feels progressively noble, delicate, and sentimental.

Why it works

- She gets a conceivably orgasmic G-spot rub from his penis as it slides against the front mass of her vagina on each push.
- It claims to her "being taken" dreams since she needs to lie still and get him.
- He has simple access and finishes the opportunity of development since he's lying in the middle of her legs; in addition to he gets that sentiment of control.
- The way that you're not eye to eye makes it simple to enjoy a private dream.

You can tailor the situation to your disposition: make it warm and sentimental for delicate cherishing, or fun-loving and unusual for wild evenings in.

CHAPTER FIVE

KAMA'S WHEEL

Kama's Wheel is an ideal piece of a long grouping of sex positions; she can move consistently into practically any lady on-top situation from Kama's Wheel basically by lying back, driving him back, or changing her leg position. It's not high on pushing the limit, so this may be the situation wherein you sit up to enjoy a reprieve and kiss each other on the lips.

"If you see a lady hurling profound moans, with her lips getting red and her eyes moping, when her mouth half opens and her developments develop carelessly... this is the minute for coition."

Kama's wheel

Why it works

- She's focused straightforwardly over his penis, so she feels completely entered.
- He can tense and loosen up the muscles of his penis to give her a hot inward back rub;
- She can respond by crushing him with her vaginal muscles.
- You both have your hands allowed to stroke and touch each other everywhere.
- She can recline on her hands and push her hips all over him.
- You can redo this situation in the manner you like. Tantric sex fans can utilize it to postpone climax and flow sexual vitality around the body. Show-offs can do it wearing titillating interest wear. Darlings getting a charge out of a get-together can utilize it to converge in sentimental ecstasy.

Silkworm turning a cover

On the off chance that the standard evangelist position feels unreasonably steady for you, attempt its raunchier connection. The lady is progressively dynamic since she has her legs noticeable all around and wrapped firmly around him. He thinks that it's energizing since he can straightforwardly feel the quality of her craving.

Why it works

- It's a staple sex position that hits quite a few spots for him and her. The pole of his penis touches her clitoris on each push.
- He can attempt long, slow, profound strokes or prodding shallow ones.
- She can utilize the intensity of her thigh muscles to pummel him in quick on each push.
- It's anything but difficult to change the sensations and the profundity of infiltration; she raises or brings down her legs. Analysis to perceive what works for you.
- If you both hold tight, you can turn more than 180 degrees into a lady on-top position.

The transformed grasp

A lady should "place her man recumbent on the bed or rug, mount his individual, and fulfill her wants," as per the antiquated writings. The Inverted Embrace isn't extraordinary for fulfilling wants, but on the other hand, it's useful for getting very close and personal.

Why it works

- With her knees propped on the bed, she can knock, protuberance, and granulate her approach to climax.
- He's allowed to lie back and watch her in execution mode, and at her hottest.
- You can luxuriate in the closeness of full-body contact and surrender yourselves to kissing and snuggling; previously, during, and after.
- It's incredible when he's worn out, and she's brimming with vitality. However, don't be surprised if he marvelously makes recuperation.

- If he's come and she hasn't, she can benefit as much as possible from the last snapshots of his erection.

Beating on the spot

Beating on the Spot was considered by a portion of the old sex masters to be the position that conveyed the most fulfillments. It is positively delicate if somewhat limiting. On the off chance that you discover you can't move as uninhibitedly as you need, appreciate the mounting feeling of sexual strain.

Why it works
- She's situated legitimately over his penis, so she feels altogether filled, and he feels capably encased.
- Your upstanding, snuggling position makes you feel strongly fortified.
- He appreciates the sensation and sight of her bosoms stroking his face.
- You experience heavenly interior tinglings as she vacillates her vaginal muscles against his pole, and he flexes his penis accordingly.
- He can put his hands under her butt to move her here and there or to and fro.

The pair of tongs

The Pair of Tongs is a staple situation in many sweethearts' sexual experiences for the basic explanation that it feels awesome for both you. To pay tribute to its name, she should utilize her vaginal muscles to grasp his part as hard as a couple of tongs.

Why it works
- The Pair of Tongs is one of the most well-known situations for ladies to arrive at the climax as there is a lot of clitoral rubbing.
- He has his hands free so that he can zest things up with some innovative craftsmanship on her bosoms, clitoris, butt, or thighs.
- As she crushes her vaginal muscles, the constrictions give him a seriously sensual sensation.
- She's in finished control of the development.
- He will adore the view from underneath.

- She can transform sex into an arousing treat by inclining forward and kneading him.

The person who stops at home

This position gives you a convincing motivation to stop at home. The sexual air snaps as she moves with liquid undulations or quick hip flicks. Close the blinds, remove each other's garments, toss yourselves on the bed, and appreciate an uproarious night in.

Why it works
- She can prod him by taking him to the verge with quick hip rascals, at that point backing things off with moderate pelvic circles.
- She can brush her hands softly at the edges of his body to make him shiver.
- He feels solid and predominant; however, she gets a kick from being the prime mover.
- She adds to the suggestive force by looking at him as she goes all over.
- If she gets worn out, you can enjoy a fast reprieve in the teacher position.

The eleventh stance

This slight bend on the evangelist position is the ideal all-rounder for various temperaments of cherishing. It's extraordinary for fulfilling unexpected sex desires and snapshots of outrageous desire, and it likewise works for long, slow, languid love when time is no item.

Why it works
- Her feet on the backs of his legs give him an unusual caught sensation.
- She can slide her feet all over his legs to change the profundity of infiltration.
- It's sentimental, personal, and warm; you can kiss, press your bodies to close and feel associated.
- You fit together superbly, and it's anything but difficult to discover a cadence that flames up both of you.

- Both of your bodies are agreeable and upheld, so you can remain in the situation for quite a while, and desert yourselves to joy en route.

Parting the bamboo

Parting the Bamboo is a sexual execution craft that meets yoga exercise. She lies on her back and lifts every leg thus all through sex. This gives him an unobtrusive however suggestive back rub as her vagina moves around his penis. It's likewise a turn-on for him on the off chance that he cherishes the sight and vibe of her legs against him. Assuming this is the case, she ought to play out her moves with expertly moderate unseemliness.

Why it works
- Each time she raises and brings down her legs, her vagina moves around his penis, which changes the interior sensations for both of you. She feels pressure on the two sides of her vagina. He feels as if his penis is by and large tenderly moved inside her.
- It allows her to play out some sexual aerobatic exhibition to an incredibly open group of spectators, and to get some extremely cozy and direct appreciation.
- Her leg positions give him the sexual vibe of being permitted in, yet kept down.
- Although he's on top, she's the one making the moves. She appreciates igniting his longing, while he appreciates the titillation of watching her.
- It's incredible if he's the near climax because the unpretentious penis knead he's getting can pull him once more from the very pinnacle of excitement.

Upheld congress
This position is made for when you're moving together at a gathering and desire beats you. You sneak off to your host's small washroom/sweeper storage room, and she squeezes him against the divider. Before you know it, she has her leg around his midriff, and you're in Supported Congress.

Why it works

- As long as your private parts are stature adjusted, he can make an abrupt exciting passage. If she's somewhat shorter than him, he can have a go at crouching to redress.
- Even on the off chance that he can't infiltrate, he can rub his penis against her clitoris.
- Supported Congress is quick and rash, and it makes you feel inconceivably provocative.
- If you're upset in an open spot, it's anything but difficult to get off, alter your garments, and set up your reasons or escape.
- If you're doing it at home, it's a perfect situation to pretend.

The stopperage

Next time you have intercourse, get a few pads from the couch and slip them under her rear end. This will raise her pelvis high and produce brilliant sensations for both of you. Indeed, after The Stopperage, you'll take a gander at pads in an entirely different light.

Why it works

- Her pelvis is raised by at least one pad, so it's simple for him to slide into her, and the point of infiltration is a champ.
- Her vagina is contracted because her knees are attracted up to her chest. This makes a phenomenally tight fit among you.
- She can slip her fingers between her legs on the off chance that she needs extra clitoral incitement.
- Although you don't have the full body to get in touch with, you can appreciate a lot of eye to eye closeness.
- You get sentiment joined with extreme suggestive sensation.

Dog and mouse sharing a gap

This is an enduring most loved for the two people. She cherishes it because the opportunity of development regularly promises her a climax. He cherishes it since he gets the chance to observe her satisfaction close-up. Also his penis profits by all the great work she's doing on top.

Why it works

- She can point herself for most extreme joy: if the leader of his penis hits the front mass of her vagina, it rubs her G-spot; if it rubs against the back divider, it invigorates her PS-spot (PS means "perineal wipe," a delicate region just underneath her perineum).
- Sustained grating between her clitoris and his pubic bone (or his abs, if he's been working out) can make this position super-climactic for her.
- It's delicate from the start, working to a hot crescendo.
- He can fulfill his desire by snatching her rear end and moving her in tight circles over him.

Sex from behind

This back section position has a similar rich sexiness, closeness, and skin-to-skin contact that you'd get if you were confronting one another, yet the way that you do not make it a touch naughtier. As consistently with back passage sex, the feeling of obscurity can be exciting

Why it works

- The front mass of her vagina gets prodded on each push, so her G-spot is altogether animated each time he moves.
- He encounters the delight of profound infiltration in addition to warm and sexy skin contact along the front of his body.
- She can sink joyfully into the bed as he encompasses her in a caring full-body grasp.
- If you're into pretend, she can be the honest virgin enticed as she lies in her bed.
- This position is perfect for both vaginal and butt-centric sex, and it feels better than being on every one of the fours.

Enormous winged animal over a dull ocean

If she's generally the one to call the sexual shots, attempt this situation wherein he's plainly in control. After some delicate enchantment, he fixes her with an evil flash in his eye, moves in with exactness precision, and dives his colossal feathered creature into her dim ocean.

Why it works

- Her legs are generally open, so he can touch her clitoris with the tip of his penis before making a fantastic, clearing passage.
- She can lie back, let go, and trust him to make the moves.
- You each have inverse jobs, which increase the sexual strain. She's detached and defenseless; he's dynamic and savage.
- He hangs over her body; however, it doesn't swarm her, which is ideal for the supported eye to eye connection straight up to climax.
- Her hands are free so that she can put them to great use on herself or him.

The frog

This is an attempt it-and-see position. Contingent upon your fabricate and adaptability, he may battle to draw near enough to enter. If you can't make it work, it's simple for her to get up and straddle him. On the off chance that it works: congrats. You've aced one of the trickier sex places of the East.

Why it works

- Because he can't enter her easily, you have to liaise intently in accomplishing the position. This is extraordinary for beating timidity and becoming more acquainted with one another (if you didn't as of now).
- Because you can't push in and out, you'll have the attractive undertaking of testing to discover novel methods for moving.
- It's warm and material; you must choose the option to hold tight to one another.
- It's conservative, so you can do it in spaces where sex would some way or another be outlandish (the storeroom/the washroom/the vehicle).

The congress of the elephant

Two mating elephants may not be your concept of suggestive paradise, yet this creature motivated position is shockingly attractive and can convey shivering G-spot sensations for her. Attempt it when she feels compliant, and he needs to assume the prevailing job.

Why it works

- His penis hits her G-spot decisively on each stroke. This expands her opportunity of having a touchy vaginal climax.
- He can look down and get the pornography style rush of seeing his penis siphoning in and out.
- She appreciates the suggestive powerlessness of being taken from behind.
- He can move unreservedly because her backside pads his pushes.

You can't see each other's countenances, so it's anything but difficult to forsake your restraints and focus on unadulterated joy.

CHAPTER SIX

PASSIONATE ADVENTURES

On the off chance that your desire is kicking like a wild pony, you're in the correct spot; these positions are expected to jog you and your sweetheart directly to the end goal. Attempt positions, for example, the Tiger Step and Late Spring Donkey when you're super-hot and unquenchable. Disregard the standards about foreplay; toss each other on the bed and continue ahead with it.

Sprinkled all through the part are some increasingly quiet positions, which are similarly exceptional however not all that requesting on the privates, hips, and pelvis. At the point when you need to focus on sensation without games, attempt stances, for example, The Lotus Position and Seagulls on the Wing.

Energetic undertakings are in every case best in new places, so take your sweetheart's hand, and drag them up and as far away as you can manage. On the off chance that your financial limit won't reach out to a five-star inn, go to the closest B&B, motel, or park seat (betrayed, obviously). In any event, make it to the extent of the washroom and do it in the shower. For a lot of different thoughts on the most proficient method to keep your energy changed, read on.

The enclosing position

The strategic maneuver of predominance and accommodation is a significant turn-on in this position. She's hitched into position on her back as he hunkers down on her, the way that she can't move except if he enables her to can be incredibly exciting for both of you.

Why it works

- She gets a show-off rush of uncovering her body as she lies with her knees attracted up to her chest.

- She's in an attractive snare that liberates her from obligation and execution pressure.
- The possibility that he's allowed to "help himself" to her body is a moment excitement sponsor.
- He gets the chance to see her in a titillating new position and from another point.
- It's a gentle method for exploring different avenues regarding subjugation sensations. There are no rope, chains, cuff, or bunches; on the off chance that you don't care for it, you unwind from the position.

The fourth stance

The front of her body is tantalizingly uncovered in this satisfyingly emotional L-formed position. This implies both of you can extravagant succulent kisses and amazing touches on every last bit of her frontal joy zones from areolas to navel, collarbone to the clitoris.

Why it works
- He controls her situation on his lap, so he can move her to a spot where he can slide effectively and profoundly into her.
- He gets an awesome perspective on her legs, tummy, bosoms, neck, and face.
- It's profoundly invigorating for both of you, yet agreeable and relaxing, so you can utilize it for adoring that is lackadaisical yet extreme.
- It's the ideal situation for her to have a mixed climax. (This is clitoral, and a G-spot climax joined.) His penis supplies the G-spot/vaginal incitement while his/her fingers chip away at her clitoris. Or then again both of you can utilize a vibrator.

The flawless stance

This is minimal sex at its raunchiest: she lies on her back with her knees attracted up to her chest, and he jumps on top and packs her with his body. It's a decent position for profound pushing, with a frisson of control to include additional experience.

Why it works

- She has next to no space to move around. Lying still is an incredible method to concentrate her psyche on sexual power.
- His amazing nearness over her is an electric turn-on if she's in a compliant mentality or needs to let him lead the pack.
- The boundary made by her legs conveys sensual erosion that he gets off on.
- He's excited by being in charge and ready to move and push uninhibitedly.
- Her hands are allowed to grasp or get his body as she draws nearer to the summit.

The goat and the tree

If she's stripping or lap moving for him, this is the perfect finale. She can prod him by revolving and twirling before him, and afterward enticingly lower herself on to his lap. Then again, he can get straight to the point and request that she comes and sits on his knee.

Why it works

- It's the ideal situation for a profoundly entering, fulfilling fast in and out.
- He adores the sheer provocativeness of being sat upon.
- If you're cautious, you can do it out in the open. She hitches up her skirt and sits down.
- It's probably the best position for her to have a hand-conveyed climax.
- He can nibble her neck and shoulder as the enthusiasm mounts.
- Providing you're not doing it on a recreation center seat, she can give him a handy exercise by the way she gets a kick out of the chance to be contacted. He essentially lays his hand over hers as she jerks off, a procedure called "hand-riding."

Lotus and Accomplishing positions

You can move flawlessly between these two positions. The Lotus Position specifically is a most loved situation for tantric sex. Attempt it when you're in the disposition for moderate lovemaking wherein suggestive sensations develop, and afterward swell all through your body.

Why they work

- In the two positions, you rock your pelvises tenderly against one another (envision you're on a shaking horse). You'll feel tasty shivering sensations extending from your privates up into your midsection.
- He's set to give loads of consideration to her bosoms and areolas.
- Being so intently laced makes an incredible enthusiastic association between you.
- The demonstration of loosening up her leg in the Accomplishing Position makes an inconspicuous, however sexy change in the fit between his penis and her vagina.

The 6th stance

All the more prevalently known as doggie style, this is a great sex position that couples regularly fall into when they're eager for basic, hair-raising sex, without decorations or sentiment. It's sex at its generally crude, fundamental, and bestial, which is actually why individuals love doing it.

Why it works

- There are no hindrances so that he can push profoundly.
- Her vaginal passageway focuses straightforwardly in reverse since she's on her knees and elbows, making this one of the most effective open situations for entrance.
- He does not just get a titillating perspective on her rear end and vulva as he enters, yet additionally appreciates the rush of watching himself push in and haul out.
- His hands are allowed to touch her back, work her bum, or stroke her rear-end.
- It feels underhanded, free, and messy, which is the thing that awe-inspiring sex is frequently about.

The substitute development of puncturing

Like the Lotus Position, this is a tantric sex exemplary. It won't convey quick and enraged beating, yet it creates an extraordinary sexual vitality that prompts mind-changing climaxes. Attempt it when you need to encounter tantric ecstasy as a primary concern, body, and soul.

Why it works

- If you rock against one another, take in synchrony, and look into one another's eyes, you'll begin to get a delightful feeling of sexual vitality developing in your pelvises.
- Your spines are straight and upstanding, so sexual vitality can travel upward from your problem areas, making rushes of sexy and sensual joy all through your bodies.
- According to tantra, she is the goddess (Shakti), and he is the god (Shiva). This position enables you to combine your manly and female substances and appreciate a euphoric and profound feeling of association.

Tiger step

The doggie position with a devious wind: rather than laying on each of the fours, in this adaptation, she brings down her head to the ground and raises her butt high noticeable all around. Sex positions don't come substantially more uncovered than this along these lines, accommodation sovereigns, appreciate it. He'll adore it in the manner he cherishes all back passage represents; it's easily messy and provocative.

Why it works

- He can press along the front mass of her vagina with each push, so her G-spot gets heaps of incitement.
- He can embed a finger into her rear-end and move it done in time with his pushes to heighten sensation for her.
- She can put her hand or a vibrator between her legs to animate her clitoris.
- If you like back passage butt-centric sex, her rear-end is effectively available for infiltration. Furthermore, butt-centric sex feels powerfully

soiled in this position. (As consistently with butt-centric sex, he ought to enter gradually and use a lot of lube).

- He gets a kick out of her posture to come and-get-me weakness.
- She appreciates giving up control and presenting herself to him.

The horse and the swing

The Mare isn't only a position; it's a system as well. "At the point when the lady coercively holds the lingam in her yoni, it is known as the Mare's Position," says the Kama Sutra. Having grasped him hard from inside, she inclines toward The Swing, one of the most sizzling back passage positions where she's in charge.

Why they work
- His penis enters her at an uncommon point. As she inclines forward into The Swing, his erection presses emphatically against the back mass of her vagina, which animates touchy spots, for example, the PS-spot (see page 94).
- In The Mare, she contracts and loosens up her vaginal muscles around his penis, so he feels tantalizingly pressed and discharged.
- He can stroke and pet her rear-end, perineum, posterior, or back.
- The perspective on her can in The Swing gets him hot. Also, he can watch his penis being provocatively encased by her.

Getting the ideal fit

A considerable lot of the situations in the Kama Sutra are proposed to make the ideal sexual fit between couples. Abnormal as it might sound, the best sexual couplings are those among stallions and elephants, bulls and horses, and rabbits and do.

The Kama Sutra partitions men into three classes of the penis: little (bunnies), medium (bulls), and enormous (stallions). Ladies aren't excluded from Vatsyayana's estimating tape: those with little, medium and huge vaginas are individually portrayed as does, female horses, and elephants.

An equivalent match

The best sex, as indicated by Vatsyayana, is between an "equivalent" couple, for instance, a bull and a female horse. In such cases, practically anything goes. Be that as it may, when the association is inconsistent, Vatsyayana trains couples to get into progressively expand positions to improve the sexual fit and make sex as fulfilling as would be prudent.

Low association

In a low association, she is greater than him. Low association combos are a bunny man and a female horse lady, or a rabbit or bull-man combined with an elephant lady. The issue with the most reduced association is an absence of sensation for both of you. She won't feel full, and he won't feel held. Vatsyayana's truly reasonable exhortation is to engage in sexual relations in The Mare's position, which is as a lot of systems as position: she gets her vaginal muscles around his penis, having been staying at work past 40 hours on her Kegel works out. Vatsyayana additionally suggests that "sex devices might be utilized"; all that anyone could need consent to whip out a vibrator or dildo from your bedside cabinet.

Different places that help in the low association are those in which she attracts her knees to her chest (to get her vagina, for example, Phoenix Playing in a Red Cave.

High association

If a lady with a little vagina engages in sexual relations with a blessed by the god's man, this is known as "high association." It sounds engaging; however, it can present issues in that his penis can, at times, feel too large for comfort. Vatsyayana acts the hero with three sex places that will "augment the yoni": Widely Opened Position, Yawning Position, and The Wife of Indra. On account of current information about female life systems, be that as it may, we realize that a portion of these positions may have the contrary impact, if a lady attracts her knees up to her chest (as in The Wife of Indra), this agreement her vagina, making it shorter.

An elective method for dealing with the potential uneasiness of high association is to ensure that a lady is super-stirred and wet before the entrance. In functional terms, this implies as a lot of foreplay as she needs and humoring her in a portion of her preferred turn-ons, regardless of whether they be cunnilingus, serious kissing, or watching him play the guitar wearing cowhand cap and chaps. When she's completely turned on (hold up until she gets to the gasping, moaning, squirming stage), she ought to be smooth with her characteristic grease, and even the biggest penis should slide in easily.

Another edge

Another method for effectively accomplishing high association is to pick sex places that limit the length of his penis or avoid him entering her completely. Anything that includes his penis pointing back through his thighs is great, for instance, Race of the Member, one next to the other positions function admirably as well, for instance, Transverse Lute or The Fifth Posture.

Yawning position

Otherwise called Legs of Victory, this position falls into the hot-enough-to-photo classification. If you extravagant yourselves as pornography stars, take a stab at videoing yourselves in Yawning Position (heels and leggings will finish the look). If you don't appreciate it for its emotional provocativeness.

Why it works
- He can animate himself (and her) with quick hip flicks so his pole siphons in and out at rapid.
- It makes her look and feel solid, supple, and super-provocative, and it's an incredible possibility for her to flaunt smooth and flawless legs, with or without tights.
- He feels like a stud as he presses all over between her legs.
- It has huge numbers of the advantages of the evangelist position (being eye to eye, having the option to push openly, etc.), yet it feels around multiple times as ignoble.

Rising position

Even though your developments are limited in this position, it rates profoundly on sexual strain since you're confronting one another, yet her legs counteract him kissing or getting excessively close. This is likewise probably the best position for giving her a pre-coital climax.

Why it works

- He can make her stop by grasping his penis and surrounding the tip on her clitoris. He would then be able to make an energizing passageway by entering her while she's in the last throes of climax, firing up her for the following one.
- He feels the sexual energy of pushing against the obstruction of her raised legs. He can likewise utilize her legs to clutch as he pushes.
- He has a titillating perspective all over, neck, and bosoms. It's additionally simple for him to contact her bosoms with his hands.
- You can up the enthusiastic force by holding each other to have a look.

The ninth stance

Think about this as the extravagance end of the doggie-position advertise; he bows upstanding behind her, and she wraps her top half over a bed or couch. You're agreeable, loose, and flawlessly situated to surrender yourselves to exceptional delight.

Why it works

- He can push profoundly and openly, and her G-spot gets bunches of incitement as he moves.
- You can make your most out of control climax face safe in the information that nobody can see.
- Unlike other doggie-style positions, she doesn't need to help her body weight on her hands or elbows; this makes for the loosened up back section, with all the standard sensuality and dream potential that doggie offers.

- If he needs to make an indirect access entrance, he's ready to do as such. Also, the way that she's agreeable will assist her with relaxing her butt-centric muscles and let him in.

Seagulls on the wing

This one will verify bunches of boxes for both of you. You don't need to be super-supple or gym fit, and, giving he's at the correct stature, the edge of section produces dangerous sensations. You can likewise put your hands to a lot of good use. The main thing you can't do is kiss.

Why it works
- The precision section gives both of you a sharp rush right now of entrance.
- She can have a mid-sex climax from some clitoral handwork (self-conveyed or from him).
- The opportunity to siphon, push, rub, and rotate can drive both of you to a quick climax.
- You have the vast majority of the advantages of a face-to-face, the man-on-top situation with the reward that he's actually in the middle of her thighs and can sink into her effectively and profoundly.
- He can get, stroke, and touch her sides, bosoms, and thighs, and she can change her areolas and stroke her bosoms.

Level feet and Raised feet stances
These two positions originate from a class called "uttana-bandha" or "prostrate stance." The old writings being nothing if not thorough, there are nine different varieties highlighted, in which the lady puts her legs in various positions.

Why they work
- In the Level Feet Posture, you can both touch one another while he moves delicately inside her; your desire increments continuously.
- She loosens up her legs provocatively as the sexual pressure increments.

- When you need increasingly lively development, move into the Raised Feet Posture; since he inclines toward his hands, he can move all the more openly and profoundly to take you both to the pinnacle.
- If she needs increasingly clitoral incitement to accomplish peak, she can reach through her legs and stroke herself to climax

Trade of coition

Tired of him being on top in the minister position? She can commandingly oust him, so he's lying level on his back with his legs spread while she jumps on top in the customarily manly half push-up. Consider it a sexual overthrow.

Why it works
- Her legs are as one, which delivers a satisfyingly cozy fit among you.
- She makes sparkles fly for both of you by snapping her pelvis quickly to and fro. This impersonates the siphoning activity of his penis.
- She can pull things again from the edge with tempting ladylike developments, for example, slow hip circles.
- There's little weight on him to perform; he needs to lie back.
- He adores seeing her over him and the impression of her bosoms stroking his chest as she moves.

Driving the peg home

Save this situation for snapshots of fabulous energy. It's energizing, widespread, and quick. For a definitive in unconstrained kicks, do it anyplace that is not at home. Reasonable settings incorporate the extra room at a gathering, a left passageway, an office (night-time), a calm backstreet, or a fix of confined forest (pick a tree that won't brush her back).

Why it works
- She feels completely infiltrated as he drives his peg home.
- The divider, despite her good faith, underpins and settles the situation as he pushes.

- If you're close to a bed, you can utilize this situation as an attractive method of transport. At the point when you land at the bed, he can bring down her on to the sleeping cushion, and afterward jump on top.
- She cherishes, feeling cleared away by the power and quality of his enthusiasm.
- He adores feeling incredible and in charge.
- It gives you the rush of just-can hardly waits for one-second energy.
- If there's even a little probability of being gotten, this adds to the feeling of prurient and mischievous earnestness.

Phoenix playing in a red cavern

This position sounds flavorful Eastern, suggestive, and colorful. Cheerfully, it satisfies its name as far as a sensation by permitting profound, extreme entrance. He feels sucked (in a larger number of ways than one) as she attracts her knees to her chest, a definitive "enter" signal.

Why it works
- Her vagina is contracted, so she feels each sensation perfectly. This position is useful for couples with low association.
- Her clitoris is uncovered, so it's a perfect situation for top-up clitoral incitement with his fingers or a sex toy.
- He appreciates physical boundary-free entrance and can dive profoundly.
- Apparent defenselessness meets sexual power as she raises her legs for him in a private sexual greeting.
- He can give her liquefying sensations by stroking the backs of her thighs.

Squeezed and Half-squeezed positions

The sensuality of these two positions originates from the blend of obstruction and consistency; the way that you're pushing against one different makes an encitingly suggestive battle. What's more, notwithstanding the way that he's in a prevailing position, she can utilize her legs to push him away in a second.

Why they work

- Pressed Position feels tight and conservative; she pushes against him with her feet, and he pushes back with his pushes.
- Her knees are pressed firmly against her bosoms, which abbreviates her vagina.
- You can both utilize your hands to knead each other's thighs (or, in case you're engaging in sexual relations that are excessively wild and uncontained for a rub, you can squeeze, get, and slap).
- Switching from Pressed to Half-Pressed Position changes the pressure with which her vagina grasps his penis; if this feels better, you can continue doing it with interchange legs.

Refined position

This is exactness sex: her vagina is inverse his penis as he bows upstanding. Accordingly, he can float in and out like a bit of well-oiled apparatus, and the smooth, customary, cadenced redundancy should take both of you directly to sex paradise.

Why it works

- Sex feels easily pleasurable because her pelvis is raised to the ideal tallness.
- His entrance is smooth and smooth.
- He can push with wild forsake or delicate limitation, contingent upon her disposition.
- She feels serenely upheld in an all the way open, prepared to-get his position.
- He can bolster each swing of his pelvis by holding her abdomen or hips.

- Four hands easily take care of animating her bosoms and clitoris to carry her to a phenomenally rapid peak.

The tenth stance

Attempt this position when you need deafening sex that takes steps to conquer you or when there's gigantic sexual strain stewing beneath the surface. It's extraordinary for releasing your feelings, tossing each other on the bed, and hammering your bodies into one another.

Why it works
- No-holds-banned, sleeping cushion beating sex is amazing and freeing for both of you.
- It's an extraordinary pressure diffuser; in case you're feeling baffled or touchy, wild sex goes about as a fantastic pressure buster.
- The headboard goes about as a prop and a safeguard, which enables you to move as openly as you need.
- You need to imaginatively devise a method for pushing and pulling against one another.
- Afterward, he can fall close to her, and you can nestle each other realizing that all your enthusiasm and vitality has been spent

The vast position

Even though "vast" probably won't fire your suggestive creative mind, the lady's fully open legs and enticingly brought hips to make sex up in this position profoundly entering and satisfying? She feels tight and attractive, and he feels masculine and in charge.

Why it works

- He can hold her around the midsection and destroy her solidly on to him.
- He feels firmly grasped by her thighs.
- She can reach up to stroke his face or snatch his hair in the throes of enthusiasm.
- She can take a turn at moving by pushing down through her feet and moving her hips.
- He can dive in right for that pleasurable, overwhelmed feeling.
- She can curve her back to drive her bosoms out; she feels provocative and dazzling, and he appreciates taking in the view.

Orgasmic job inversion

"Permitting" the lady a turn on top was suggested for events when a man was "never again equipped for a solid effort." Fortunately, a lady no longer needs to hold up until her darling is limp and latent to attempt this position—she can bounce on top at whatever point she likes.

Why it works

- She's responsible for her pleasure; she can stroke off with him inside her, she can squat and push, she can circle her hips, or she can sit still and relish the association.
- He can lie there and experience the attractive delight of being utilized and manhandled.
- If she has solid thighs, she can bounce all over on the tip of his penis for a couple of strokes, and afterward lower herself to encase the entire of his pole. Visit reiteration of this method should take him to breaking point.
- He gets an incredible perspective on her squirming and agitating over him.

Turning

This is great from the Kama Sutra lobby of acclaim; you can't guarantee Kama Sutra's sexpert status except if you've done it (or endeavored it) at any rate once. It begins in a standard man-on-top position - everything looks OK - yet then he finishes a 180-degree turn so he winds up snuggling her toes. Furthermore, if that isn't sufficiently precarious, he should remain inside her for the span of the turn

Why it works

- It's one of those curiosity positions you can gloat about a while later.
- She addresses the difficulty of keeping him erect not by outer developments, however, by being lustful and intriguing.
- You both find energizing new sensations and points of entrance.
- His glans and shaft press against the sides of her vagina (ordinary sex, for the most part, includes penile weight on simply the front and back vaginal dividers)
- If he effectively finishes the turn, he's qualified to challenge her to do the comparable.

Keeping it shifted

As the old writings state, it is the "need of shifted delights" that drives darlings to the grasps of outsiders. So don't hold up until recognition and repetitiveness set in, keep the sexual pressure popping between you regularly by accepting each conceivable open door to be wicked.

It's workable for sweethearts to see each other consistently and rest together consistently without really taking a gander at one another. Keeping it fluctuated will compel you to sit up and notice your accomplice, however extravagant, fetishize, and salivate over them.

Flaunting Exhibitionism can mean coolly twisting around without any undies on, or serving supper wearing only a pooch neckline. If you don't consider yourself a characteristic big cheese, pursue these tips:

- Maximize your positive focuses. If you have sexy legs, feature them with leggings.
- Do a striptease, with your preferred music as support to give you a certainty help.
- Treat your darling to an enticing lap move.
- Radiate sexual certainty and give your sweetheart an underhanded grin. This beats an ideal body unfailingly.

Accessorise

In case you're sex toy-timid, it merits looking into your frame of mind. Once in awhile but well-disposed dots or G-spot dildos are actually what you have to land yourself a stupendously mind-bowing climax. (Even though does take note of that anything that goes up anybody's butt must have a flared base.) Even the Kama Sutra prescribes decorating sex, after a design; men can either wear penis rings or add objects into openings pierced in the penis. The mystery of getting a charge out of sex toys is to utilize them on one another (instead of in isolation) and to add them to your sexual coexistence as you'd add fixings to an incredible dinner. Pick them cautiously, and use them sparingly. They're there to improve as opposed to overwhelming your menu (and they're positively not there to camouflage the way that something's not working).

Battery-controlled sex

It might be the way that a toy focuses on your clitoral head/G spot/P-spot with logical exactness, or that a sex toy doesn't get worn out like your sweetheart's hand or it might just be that frisson of deviousness that turns you on like nothing else. Whatever the explanation, vibrators can put the gracious my-God once more into sex. Sex-toy learners: start with a straightforward, nitty-gritty vibrator and use it on his problem areas just like hers.

Anyplace yet the room

On the off chance that you return to your juiciest recollections, odds are they are of sex that occurred outside the room: that time you did it on a swing, a recreation center seat, a twilight seashore, in the lunchroom at work, or up a mountain. Your way of life (also the law) may not allow you to shag in peculiar or intriguing areas; however, you can stir up your sexual coexistence basically by attempting a no-sex-in-the-room arrangement. Be inventive.

Crazy

Some of the time, it's great to change character during sex. This is the place pretend in: you can surrender your gentle habits and become a dominatrix, or quit being the jeans-wearing chief and comply with like a startled little dog. Since you're abruptly free from your ordinary content, you can alternately identify with your accomplice and, the best part is that you have an alternate sort of sex. You don't have to set up muddled situations for pretend; you can essentially wear an outfit that you wouldn't typically wear.

The fitting on of the sock

Her clitoris is solidly middle of everyone's attention in this lady on-top position. Before he infiltrates, he takes his penis solidly in his grasp and uses it as a vibrator around her clitoral hood. At that point, when she's wet and squirming, he dives in to do some inside work.

Why it works

- If she doesn't originate from intercourse alone, this position is perfect for top-up incitement. He grasps his pole and flicks his glans back and forth over her clitoris (he can do this both previously and during sex).
- He turns into a world-class individual from the cliterati; by utilizing his penis as a sex toy, he adapts precisely what sort of pace, weight, and cadence she needs to arrive at the climax.
- He gets the opportunity to appreciate sex with her when she's at breaking point; her extraordinary excitement will be super-irresistible, particularly if she tells him how turned on she is.

Pre-summer jackass

If you think your sexual coexistence is excessively clean as a whistle, you can utilize the graceless Late Spring Donkey to sex things up. It's basic, bestial, and mischievous, and there's no space for habits, sentiment, or amenability, which can now and then be actually what you need.

Why it works

- It's crude and prepared straightforward sex; you'll both love its twist around and slip-it-in promptness.
- She gets a surge from being beat from behind while the blood races to her head.
- If she's G-spot-delicate, the drumming on the front mass of her vagina can prompt a body-convulsing G-spot climax.
- A well-coordinated hit on her bum will give her a shock of unexpected joy.
- She can attempt another move: quickly shaking her legs while he remains still. The vibes will resonate all through your bodies.

Corresponding sights of the back

Additionally referred to in the exchange as "I'll show you my mine on the off chance that you'll show me yours," this is a novel method for gazing at one another's under locales. He lifts his head to see the split of her bottom provocatively roosted over him. She, in the interim, inclines forward to see his rear end and his balls, however the provocative display of his penis diving into her.

Why it works

- If she loves pornography style close-ups, she's scored the best seat in the house.
- If both of you like pornography style close-ups, she can video the activity from where she's sitting. Watch the recording back subsequently, and end up getting horny once more.
- He can get all worked up by seeing her butt rising and falling on his paunch.
- Her rear end spread out as she settles firmly against him; the outcome is hot grinding between her perineum and his mid-region.
- She gets the opportunity to make the moves: long, smooth here and their strokes, inward constrictions, or squirms that bring his penile head into an ideal arrangement with her G-spot.
- You're in your different universes, so you can make your contemplations as scratch and dent section grimy as you like.

The winged serpent turn & Galloping horse

The intrigue of this fiery pair of positions lies in the sensual air they make as much as the careful situation of your appendages. Let the state of mind consume from seething force to thundering flares of energy as you both jog toward the end goal.

Why they work

- She's excited by the manner in which he weighs down ravenously as though he can hardly wait another minute.
- He's inebriated by the "I need you presently" non-verbal communication of her all the way open legs and the manner in which her heels pull him in profound.
- You can both close your eyes and relish the joy of a profound association, both physical and passionate.

Moving from The Dragon Turn to Galloping Horse ups the predominance/accommodation stakes. She uncovers her trust in him as she lets him "hold her down" at the foot and neck. He gets the Spanish fly intensity of having her totally in his grasp.

CHAPTER SEVEN

EROTIC EXPERTISE

The situations in this section are, for the most part, scorchingly hot, profoundly troublesome, or uncontrollably unsanitary. You'll discover a portion of the antiquated world's most noteworthy desire quenchers here nearby probably the best sexual masterpieces if watching yourselves is a turn-on, presents an ideal opportunity to set up a tripod and camcorder.

The majority of these positions expect sweethearts to be low on restraint and high on adaptability. What's more, some rely upon him being huge in the biceps office. Attempt stances, for example, Suspended Congress after he's had a couple of sessions at the rec center and Tail of the Ostrich after she's been to yoga. On the other hand, sensual mastery can mean realizing when to swindle. There's no disgrace in letting her hands, his back, or she can lean against a convenient divider or tabletop.

At long last, when you've Hung the Bow, Raced the Member, Fixed the Nail, and Spun the Top, you can lie back and take a merited break. Gather the remainder of your vitality and go as far as possible of the part for the best in post-sex comedowns.

Suspended congress

This is wild one-night-stand material. Your central goal is to attempt the most smoking, trickiest, showiest positions known to man and lady, and Suspended Congress checks all the containers. Your point: to end your sex session winded, moist, and 100 percent satisfied.

Why it works
- Its sex at its generally vivacious: she feels like a sex sovereign; he feels like a sex god. What's more, it's optimal for remembering your youthfulness.

- You needn't bother with a bed; any little work area or void divider space will do.
- It humors her jolt of energy and-hold-me-in your-arms dreams. Furthermore, on the off chance that he pulls it off, he can loll in that I'm-so-solid inclination.
- If this is the first time when you engaged in sexual relations with one another, this will break the ice and make you amazingly acquainted with each other. The main test will be what limits are breaking position to attempt straightaway.

Position of equivalents and the snake trap

Try not to be deceived by the simple and cordial appearance of these two situations, as they aren't what they appear. There's a fuming snake pit of sensation happening in that spot in your laps, so spread yourselves in knead oil and squirm like snakes.

Why they work

- His vicinity to her bosoms gives him a sensual eyeful and an areola snacking significant piece.
- An ordinary in-and-out push is practically inconceivable, so you're constrained into some wiggly shrewdness.
- Things get off to a fun-loving beginning as she sits in his lap, at that point get saucier as you move into The Snake Trap and verify each other's legs in an iron grasp that says, "I'm not giving up."
- Enjoy the tussle-like nature of The Snake Trap; squirming against one another is ensured to free you of sexual pressure

The tail of the ostrich

In case you're one of those folks who like to be a transcending nearness during sex, this is perfect. Also, if she loves being topsy turvy while scaling his pinnacle, you're an ideal counterpart for one another. The single word of alert: this isn't generally reasonable for after-supper skips.

Why it works

- He can focus on his pole parallel movement against her vulva to fill her with softening margarine sensations.
- You get the opportunity to stare at one another from an altogether new point.
- Her legs-together position makes tight waves of joy for both of you.
- He can explore different avenues regarding a novel sexual other option: diving his ostrich tail to and fro between her fastened thighs. He can either make this the headliner or a shocking opener. In any case, scouring some lube on her thighs will make this his new sexual safe house.

Lotus-like

Here's another piece of Kama Sutra tumbling to make you hot and sweat-soaked (much more so in case you're not a world-class yogi). If you can't do a lotus position, cheat by folding your legs; the impact is a lot of the equivalent. On the off chance that you can deal with the lotus: regard.

Why it works

- He can't plumb her profundities; however, the tip of his penis bumps her vaginal passageway in the most tempting manner. This develops your animalistic hunger to the point where you're prepared to eat up one another.
- The boundary of her tied legs gives you springy, fun sensations you won't get in some other sex position.
- You can praise each other for having super-propelled sex.
- It's ideal for ace/slave pretending games; with her legs sandwiched between you, there's little possibility of a simple getaway

The hanging bow

Her body bends from his at a disturbing edge in this aerobatic position for adaptable sweethearts. Before you state an apprehensive "No chance," pause for a minute to think about the curiosity, and the colossal post-coital pomposity that anticipates you on the off chance that you do figure out how to pull it off. Moreover, it's ensured to make you the visitors of respect at any sex party

Why it works

- The sheer challenge shows you a significant level of sexual cooperation; on the off chance that you can effectively accomplish The Hanging Bow, your sexual coexistence knows no limits.
- You get a sensual buzz from the extended physicality of the position.
- All the blood races to her head, giving her an eye-popping regular high.
- Being topsy turvy is beneficial for you; as indicated by reversal lovers, it supports flow, eases the pressure, empowers great stance, eases back and neck torment, diminishes balding and expands adaptability. Some state that every day reversal even encourages you to age nimbly

Matched feet

With its bizarre edge of the entrance, this is the lawn chair of sex positions: it's laid-back and uniquely crafted for relaxing sex on a blistering summer's day, ideally by the poolside. Attempt it while lying back and tasting a Screaming Orgasm or a Sex on the Beach.

Why it works

- She shudders and waves her vaginal muscles to give him a growing tide of joy.
- She lies back on her elbows with a come-and-get-me easygoing quality that attracts him.
- It's incredible for displaying her bosoms and making him discombobulated with want.
- It's tight and minimized, making it ideal for packed desire in loungers, lawn chairs, couches, and twin beds.
- Your developments are more flexing and squirming than pounding and beating. They help him to take care of business since they're unobtrusive instead of strenuous.

The third stance

It would seem that she's doing a mid-air run; however, this is a decent position for pulling him in as opposed to fleeing from him. Do it when you need all the delight and closeness of vis-à-vis adoring', yet with a scramble of extra smoothness.

Why it works

- He can get her scintillatingly moderate strokes, or he can do an abrupt pummel for sensual stun esteem.
- You're secured suggestive fight. He pushes against her thigh, trying to draw nearer. She holds firm with her leg propped against his chest. Fortunately, because it feels so hot and hot, you're the two victors.
- She can tailor it to her adaptability rating; her leg might be anything from somewhat raised to contacting her jaw.
- If he's a leg sweetheart, the smooth feel of her thigh will speed him toward the end goal.

The spouse of Indra

He stoops respectfully before her as she offers herself up in a provocative half shoulder stand. Acknowledge her idea by getting her hips and diving in. Attempt this situation after serious foreplay, when you're both at the pinnacle of excitement and prepared for some amazing sensations.

Why it works

- Her vagina is abbreviated, which makes sex feel super-exceptional for both of you, and is an advantage if he's a rabbit and she's an elephant.
- Her half shoulder stand is one of those who uncover all represent that will make him crosseyed with want.
- Her feet against his chest give her incredible influence if she needs to control the movement.
- His penis is near her butt; if you need butt-centric sex to highlight on your sexual menu, he doesn't need to go far. (For the good of hygiene, never pursue butt-centric sex with vaginal sex).

Shouting out

It looks as simple as plunking down and having a kiss; however, it's one of the most troublesome sex places of the East. The plunking down kiss is the basic piece - the test is for him to get her and swing her from side to side on his pole.

Why it works

- The pendulum-like developments on his penis will possibly send him into space.
- The bizarre plane of movement puts fulfilling pressure as an afterthought divider of her vagina.
- It improperly reveals all your me-Tarzan, you-Jane dreams.
- She cherishes being helpless before his desire.
- If you can't deal with the side-to-side swing, you can soften into euphoric eye-staring, hold-each-other-tight sex.
- You're only two or three simple developments from the cowgirl position if you need it.

Congress of the cow

Made for profane measures of desire and lewdness, this position is perfect as a feature of a prodding pretends. She twists around to "get something," he steers up behind her and, uh oh, before you know it, her skirt's around her midriff, and his jeans are embracing his lower legs.

Why it works

- The profound surge when he initially enters will make you both wheeze with delight.
- Anal sex is a choice; it feels shamefully devilish in this position.
- You're left to concentrate without anyone else delight since you're not eyeing to the eye, which is a positive in addition to if you, for the most part, give all your regard for your sweetheart's needs.
- He can get her a hot back rub that incorporates shock visits to her perineum, in addition to some hanky-panky butt cheek hitting.
- If she hasn't yet found her G-recognize, presently an extraordinary chance.

Cheerful endings

You've quite recently finished a long-distance sex race, and you're lying limp and fulfilled in one another's arms. The Kama Sutra now says: "go unobtrusively to the washing place without taking a gander at one another." Feel allowed ignoring it on this event; post-orgasmic euphoria is vastly improved mutual.

After sex, you're flooded with feel-great synthetic substances, for example, oxytocin and endorphins, which are the body's regular sedatives. These consolidate to give you a characteristic high, which is the reason it's a smart thought to lounge in this state for as long it keeps going.

Animalistic blow

Snuggle up to one another and murmur delicately. Float in the scrumptious state among rest and alertness, and zone in on all the warm, shivering postsex sensations coursing through your bodies. Stroke one another. Take the risk to pronounce your tenderest emotions

The Ananga Ranga had the correct thought; Kalyana Malla's recommendation to men was: "The point at which your desirous skips are at an end, take care not to get up tersely. Rather, delicately pull back your part and remain with your darling. Lie on your correct side in the bed of joy. Along these lines, you won't look like a man who mounts a lady like a donkey and gives no consideration to the specialty of affection."

Going around once more

The postcoital period can likewise be the point at which she has her first/second/third climax. On the off chance that she's as yet tingling with want and he's spent and limp, look for a trade-off: you can both alternate to invigorate her, or he can furnish some static vaginal entrance with his fingers while she gets down to business on her clitoris. A vibrator is likewise an incredible postcoital climax supplier. On the other hand, she can hold tight for cycle two. Contingent upon how old he is (and how drained and how inspired), the time it takes for him to get hard again might be anything from minutes to hours. The speediest method to get him back in the state of mind is a power rest, trailed by fluid refreshments, a provocative back rub, and her X-appraised proposals murmured in his ear.

Refueling

Sharing an arousing postcoital nibble is an extraordinary method to drag out the state of mind and remain in that close "we've simply engaged in sexual relations" bubble. This is particularly valid on the off chance that you share a similar tub of marginally dissolved frozen yogurt, taste from a similar glass of full-bodied red wine, or feed each other succulent grapes or strawberries with your fingers, even Vatsyayana, who debilitated postcoital eye to eye connection and sent sweethearts off to the restroom for an energetic after-sex clean, suggests postcoital holding over a beverage and a tidbit. You might need to avoid the slop, however:

"The man should grasp her with his left arm and urge her to drink from a cup that he grasps. The couple can eat sweetmeats; they can drink crisp juice, soup, slop, concentrates of meat, sherbet, the juice of mango organic product, or the concentrate of the juice of the citron tree."

Postcoital positions

Discover a place that lets you loosen up your entire body with the goal that you can savor that liquefied inclination in comfort. Spoons' position is useful for remaining nearby at the same time, for a definitive in closeness, takes a stab at folding into Side-by-Side clasping (see page 38) and squeezing your temples together. On the other hand, there's something quirkily cozy about winding up with your heads by one another's feet. Also, after strenuous, bed-breaking episodes of sex, nothing beats lying on your backs and clasping hands while smiling at the roof.

CHAPTER EIGHT

ANAL SEX

The Art of Anal Intercourse goes back to old occasions recommends that the act of butt-centric sex incitement of the anorectal zone, including penile infiltration, has been around for a long time. Some may think that it's amazing how basic training it is among hetero couples today. In one overview of 100,000 female readers of Redbook magazine, 43 percent of the ladies said they'd attempted it with their accomplices at any rate once. Of that number, 40 percent said they discovered it fairly or truly charming. (That is, about a fourth of the all outnumber of ladies reviewed said this.) Forty-nine percent said they couldn't have cared less for it, and 10 percent said they had no solid sentiments one way or the other. While not a controlled logical examination, this study generally parallels the discoveries of numerous other sexual overviews.

Something different that may come as amazement to many: While a reasonable number of heteros participate in the training, not all gay people do. In a survey of the current information regarding the matter, the Kinsey Institute presumed that somewhere in the range of 59 and 95 percent of male gay people had occupied with butt-centric sex at any rate once.

In the period of AIDS, butt-centric sex has gotten a great deal of terrible press and all things considered. Unprotected butt-centric intercourse is the absolute most dangerous conduct as far as an introduction to the feared illness. It bears referencing, notwithstanding, that if neither you nor your accomplice is as of now tainted with HIV (human immunodeficiency infection), you can't get AIDS from butt-centric sex. This may appear to be obvious, yet in an across the country sex review directed by the Kinsey Institute, half of the American grown-ups addressed said they figured you could get AIDS through butt-centric intercourse, regardless of whether one accomplice was tainted. This is false.

What is genuine is that having butt-centric intercourse with a contaminated accomplice, without utilizing a condom, is the sort of sex conduct well on the way to transmit AIDS. That is presumably because the delicate covering of the rectum is probably going to tear during intercourse, permitting AIDS-tainted blood or semen to pass straightforwardly into a sex accomplice's circulatory system. The proof for this method of AIDS transmission is so clear-and AIDS itself is terrifying to such an extent that specialists currently prescribe against having butt-centric sex with anyone, under any conditions.

If you demand to attempt it, at any rate, avoid potential risk: The vagina is normally versatile and saturated by its very own regular oils, however, the rectum isn't. Consequently, before endeavoring butt-centric infiltration, it's essential to utilize a water-based grease like K-Y Jelly. Additionally, before entering the vagina after butt-centric intercourse, makes certain to wash the penis completely. Something else, it's probably going to move microorganisms from the rectum, which may cause vaginal contaminations.

Contraception

The ovulation testing pack is a new strategy for common family arranging that enables you to appreciate having intercourse without utilizing any contraceptives on most days of your cycle. The pack incorporates an individual screen that checks your pee tests and examinations them to demonstrate the times of the month on which you are probably going to get pregnant. You should utilize contraceptives if you wish to have intercourse on those days. The pack is 93-95 percent solid and simple to utilize.

Common family arranging, on the other hand, requires careful record keeping and iron self-restraint. It includes graphing your temperature step by step all through the menstrual cycle to find the time of ovulation, during which you should refuse sex. Any capricious anomaly in the cycle can convey the danger of pregnancy.

The Pill is up to 99 percent dependable. It takes into consideration unconstrained lovemaking. The opportunity it gives is of tremendous mental advantage in any relationship. The Pill additionally controls the menstrual cycle and diminishes period agony and overwhelming seeping in numerous ladies. Mellow symptoms happen in certain ladies who take the Pill, yet they normally vanish following a couple of months. They may incorporate queasiness, cerebral pains, and misery, weight increase and some seeping between periods. If symptoms continue, the specialist or center will ordinarily prescribe a difference in contraception. Before your primary care physician endorses the Pill, the person will request your therapeutic history, remembering the frequency of thrombosis for your family. The wellbeing dangers associated with taking the Pill are slight when contrasted with the dangers of pregnancy and labor.

The joined Pill contains manufactured types of the sex hormones estrogen and progesterone, which meddle with the lady's normal 28day menstrual cycle. In a lady who isn't taking the Pill, the creation of the sex hormones varies during the cycle, and it is this change that triggers ovulation. At the point when the Pill keeps the hormone level misleadingly steady, the sign to ovulate is counteracted. The equivalent occurs during pregnancy, which is the reason covering pregnancies don't happen. Any individual who smokes vigorously might be in danger of thrombosis, smokers and the individuals who are more than 35 are regularly prompted not to take the consolidated Pill.

The progestogen - just Pill isn't, as some of the time accepted, a low portion Pill, yet one containing a solitary hormone, progestogen. It has the impact of thickening the emissions in the cervix, which makes it hard for sperm to pass. It very well may be taken by bosom sustaining moms, in contrast to the consolidated Pill, which smothers lactation.

The condom is 85-98 percent successful as a technique for contraception. Condoms work by keeping the sperm from getting to its goal, and they don't meddle with the body's science. The condom is additionally the way to safe sex as it ensures against all explicitly transmitted sicknesses. For more insights concerning condoms and how to utilize them, see page 128. Tops and stomachs go about as a preventative by framing a hindrance over the neck of the belly (cervix), which keeps the sperm from coming to and preparing the egg. A solid match is essential. You should be analyzed by your PCP or family arranging center with the goal that the right-sized top or stomach can be picked, and you can be told the best way to embed it. A top or stomach ought to consistently be utilized with a spermicide.

This blend has been seen as a 95 percent safe preventative. Smear a little spermicide on to the stomach and around the edge, to encourage addition. Crush the stomach into a pontoon shape and addition it as you would a sterile tampon, opening the lips of the vagina with one hand. At the point when the edge rests behind the pubic bone at the front and the vault covers the cervix at the back, it is set up. Specialists prescribe that you ought not to leave the stomach or top set up for longer than 24 hours, yet you should sit tight for at any rate six hours after intercourse before expelling it. Recollect that spermicide will be viable just for around three hours, so you should place more into the vagina on the off chance that you have sex after the stomach or top has been set up for that time. At the point when you expel the stomach or top, wash it cautiously in warm lathery water and enable it to dry in a warm spot, or pat delicately with a towel.

The female condom is as powerful as other hindrance techniques. It lines the vagina and has an internal ring that sits over the cervix and an external ring that falsehoods level against the labia. The female condom is made of vapid scentless polyurethane. The lady drives the condom up inside her vagina before intercourse, and subsequently expels it and discards it. Like the male condom, the female condom isn't reusable. It comes prepared greased up for simple addition, and no spermicide is essential. Female condoms are made in one size just and will fit all ladies. During intercourse, it is a smart thought for the lady to manage the man's penis into the condom to ensure it doesn't enter the vagina outside the condom. As the female condom is baggy, it will move during sex; however, you will, in any case, be ensured, because the penis remains inside the condom. To expel the condom after sex, turn the external ring to keep the semen inside, and haul the condom out tenderly.

The I U D (intra-uterine gadget) or loop is a little plastic and copper gadget that is embedded into the belly to counteract origination. Just a specialist prepared in family arranging can do this. The IUD comes compacted in a slender cylinder, which is slid through the cervical trench into the uterus and afterward pulled back, leaving the IUD to spring into shape. Slight strings dangle from the IUD about 3cm/1 inch into the vagina, and these can be felt with the fingers to ensure that the gadget is still set up. To expel an IUD, the specialist pulls strings with an uncommonly planned instrument.

Contingent upon the type, IUDs are normally supplanted about at regular intervals. The IUD is figured to be 96-99 percent viable as a prophylactic, even though it isn't clear precisely how it functions. Numerous ladies like it since it enables the two accomplices to be unconstrained in their lovemaking. Be that as it may, it sometimes falls short for everybody. A few ladies experience inconvenience and seeping for a couple of hours or days after the IUD is embedded, and one out of four ladies must have it expelled as a result of intense agony and substantial dying. Some of the time, an IUD may drop out; this is bound to occur during a period than at some other time, and this is the reason it is imperative to check consistently that the flimsy strings are still inside the vagina.

Prophylactic infusions might be given with a medication that contains hormones of the progestogen type. An infusion is required every 8-12 weeks and is essentially 100 percent solid prophylactics. Be that as it may, it regularly disruptively affects a lady's menstrual cycle, making periods progressively visit or even vanish out and out. Return of customary periods might be deferred for as long as a year after the last infusion.

Prophylactic inserts discharge a hormone into the circulatory system. The inserts are little, stick-like, and malleable. They are embedded under the skin of the internal upper arm by your primary care physician or facility in a straightforward, nearly torment free system. They can't be seen. The impacts will keep going for as long as five years, and even though the inserts can be expelled whenever the body won't be free of the hormone for a brief span after that. Inserts are more than 99 percent dependable, even though they may make periods less ordinary or vanish by and large. These reactions may settle down following a while.

Crisis contraception is likewise called a 'next day contraceptive.' This final hotel strategy can be utilized if intercourse has occurred without contraception or if the standard technique has fizzled, a state in case of a burst condom. It might likewise be endorsed to a lady after a rape. It very well may be offered as long as 72 hours after intercourse and is 96-99 percent successful.

The threat of AIDS, youngsters frequently had intercourse with another accomplice without a condom, especially on the off chance that they had been drinking. Remember that AIDS is significantly more risky to your wellbeing than pregnancy, and not at all like pregnancy, it's impossible that the sickness can be ended. The message is clear: any individual who takes part in easygoing sex or is having intercourse with another accomplice should utilize a condom regardless of whether the Pill gives preventative insurance. Ladies, just as men, are prescribed to convey condoms with them.

Clean bodies are commonly more engaging than grimy ones; however, the smell of a darling's perspiration can have sexual enhancer characteristics. Washing isn't constantly practicable or attractive; however, you ought to consistently wash the private parts and butt before sex, to ensure against contamination, to build the delight in your accomplice and to give fearlessness. Cleanser and water are for the most part that is required. Antiperspirants and fragrances murder the body's awesome regular aromas, and they add taste disagreeable. Vaginal antiperspirants can be decidedly destructive, pulverizing the smaller scale living beings in the vagina that ensure against ailment. Continuously wash whatever is embedded in the butt, as butt-centric sex conveys the most elevated danger of disease.

Female climax

Since the 1960s, when Kinsey started to bring sex out of the storage room, there has been such a lot of open discourse fixated on the female climax that numerous ladies feel under extraordinary strain to 'perform.' If you feel your accomplice is contrasting you with past darlings, or to an orgasmic perfect in his mind, it degrades the close joy of sex and transforms it into a challenge.

Numerous ladies are pestered by the possibility that there might be two kinds of climax - vaginal and clitoral. They wonder whether the climaxes they are encountering are 'the genuine article.' Be that as it may, are there extremely two sorts of climax? It was Freud who initially recommended that there were. He said that the climax experienced through clitoral incitement was the forerunner of a more profound, additionally fulfilling climax experienced in the vagina during entrance by the penis. As per him, the vaginal climax was a 'genuine, develop' sexual reaction, while the clitoral climax was its juvenile second rate. The worth decisions Freud and his adherents set on the two kinds of climax have caused a ton of misery among certain ladies who never experience climax during infiltration. They feel that they are passing up a major opportunity, and are in this manner insufficient: not exactly 'genuine ladies.'

Specialists into sexual reaction have been abundantly worried about the order of the female climax since Freud's time. Kinsey's view was that there was just one sort of climax, that it was activated by clitoral incitement and included constrictions of all pieces of the female body, including the vagina. He couldn't recognize the second sort of climax that focused exclusively on the vagina, and he invalidated Freud's differentiation among 'develop' and 'youthful' climaxes.

Resulting clinical proof has demonstrated convincingly that Kinsey was correct, and now sexologists have commonly concurred that a climax is a climax. Specialist Helen Kaplan has arrived at this resolution: 'Paying little respect to how rubbing is applied to the clitoris, for example by the tongue, by the lady's finger or her partner's, by a vibrator, or by copulation, the female climax is likely constantly evoked by clitoral incitement. Be that as it may, it is constantly communicated by circurnvaginal muscle release.'

Albeit all climaxes are equivalent; ladies do report various sensations as indicated by whether they are being infiltrated or jerked off. What's more, the shock is that masturbatory climaxes, which are experienced by all ladies who can instruct themselves to come through masturbation, alone or with an accomplice, are the more pleasurably intense, all ladies who climax this way know the intense pressure of the clitoris, the curvy hurrying vibe that breaks into numerous constrictions of the encompassing tissue, a little minority of ladies (around 20 percent, as indicated by sex specialist Shere Hite), who likewise climax with a penis inside the vagina, depict that as a very unique encounter. Even though Freud asserted that climaxes during intercourse were unrivaled, most of the ladies in a review did by Shere Hite said they were less extraordinary. While the masturbatory climax is experienced as a high, sweet, undulating sensation, the pinnacle of affectability, climax with entrance resembles the blast of a removed blast, amazing, however, to some degree muted.

Climaxes activated by the accomplice's fingers or tongue, and by masturbation, are likely increasingly exceptional because incitement is progressively restricted and all the more delicately guided. Bosses and Johnson announced more grounded compression fits and higher paces of the heartbeat during climax without intercourse, and particularly during masturbation. Numerous ladies affirmed that they had their best climaxes when alone. Climax during entrance is without a doubt very uncommon for some ladies because a pushing penis can animate the clitoris just 'in passing,' if by any stretch of the imagination, contingent upon the situation of the couple. The climax experienced might be progressively diffuse because the penis changes the focal point of consideration from the clitoris to the entire of the lower some portion of the lady's body, and because the vagina is full 'suppressing' the sensation.

Asynchronous climax, when the two accomplices meet up during entrance, may feel like a shockingly huge underground blast, yet it presumably offers the least as far as exotic mindfulness. The explanation behind this is if the two gatherings are centered on their understanding of 'dark out' and become negligent of one another, the impression of the accomplice's climax is generally lost. For a lady, a synchronous climax is regularly trailed by a sentiment of bewilderment, and a failure that lovemaking has concluded.

Climax during intercourse is frequently less intense. Be that as it may, a large number of the ladies who can encounter it incline toward it for passionate reasons, since it includes total body-to-body contact, holding the accomplice, and offering oneself to him simultaneously. Feeling like nothing is wrong with the world and adored and genuinely fulfilled are significant parts of a decent sexual relationship; however, these sentiments can be experienced whether climax happens during intercourse or not. What is significant is that ladies should encounter customary masturbatory climaxes. Climax alleviates strain, revives the body and renews the psyche. It leaves the lady feeling shimmering and entirety. At the point when imparted to an accomplice, it speaks to the pinnacle of sexual satisfaction and can be an amazing articulation of adoration, joining the couple.

Different and consecutive climaxes, as vaginal and clitoral climaxes, are ideas that have caused a ton of disarray and left numerous ladies stressed that their sexual reaction might be to some degree insufficient. Since climaxes come in waves, a few ladies are not by any means sure whether their climaxes are different or single. Various climaxes are those that are knowledgeable about a chain, one legitimately after another; consecutive climaxes are those with a hole of a couple of moments between everyone. It appears that different genuine climaxes are incredibly uncommon, albeit numerous ladies are fit for the consecutive climax.

On the subject of various climax, Masters and Johnson expressed: "If a female who is equipped for having standard climaxes is appropriately invigorated inside a brief period after her first peak, she will in many occurrences be fit for having a second, third, fourth, and even a fifth and 6th climax before she is completely satisfied. As stood out from the male's typical powerlessness to have more than one climax in a brief period, numerous females, particularly when clitorally invigorated, can routinely have five or six full climaxes inside merely minutes."

Being fit for six climaxes straight isn't equivalent to requiring or in any event, needing that many, as indicated by Shere Hite, around 90 percent of ladies who climax feel happy with a solitary peak. What's more, in numerous ladies, the clitoris stays easily affected, and further incitement is awkward and can even demonstrate excruciating.

Does the G-spot truly exist?

The G-spot is named after its pioneer, Ernst Grafenberg. While numerous ladies still uncertainty its reality, others guarantee that animating a spot about 5cm/2 creeps inside the vagina towards the front of the body gives them exceptional joy. The G-spot is said to be what might be compared to the male prostate organ, which is arranged about 5cm/2 creeps up the rectum towards the front of the body. The incitement of both these spots can prompt climax now and again. A few ladies have even discovered that they discharge a liquid on the off chance that they have a climax by incitement of the G-spot, and specialists in Canada and the United States guarantee that the creation of the liquid is surprisingly like the emission of the prostate organ.

How would you discover the G-spot?

On the off chance that you question the presence of the G-spot, you can attempt to discover it yourself, the least demanding approach to arrive at it is with your own or your accomplice's finger. Yet, there are additional positions for intercourse in which the penis invigorates the delicate region. The back section is ideal, especially with the man on top and a cushion underneath your hips, so the penis presses against the front mass of the vagina.

Homosexuality

Human sexuality is a mind-boggling wonder, and not all that conveniently classified by the marks 'hetero' and 'gay' as a society could wish. Between the solid and select fascination of man to lady, and that of man to man, or lady to lady, lies an entire range of sexual and enthusiastic affinities: the vigor, or warmth, or coolness of any human relationship relies upon the people inside it, and not on any of the subjective determinations which may be forced by society.

A few men need sex with other men as a lasting piece of their lives; some are interested about male bodies, and may test sooner or later in their lives; some vibe similarly pulled in to men and ladies; a few men appreciate taking a gander at other men's bodies without wanting sexual reach; some lean toward the organization of other men for relaxation; some work in an all-male condition. Ladies additionally feel and do every one of these things with other ladies. These vast stages and the perplexity that outcomes from them can't be obliged by society, which needs a request in which to work. The request implies overlooking differing shades of dim and recognizing just among highly contrasting; it implies putting names on things. What's more, since society is never more grounded than when it is joined against a typical insidiousness, marking things likewise implies characterizing society's pariahs.

Different endeavors have been made this century to 'clarify' homosexuality, and even to 'fix' it. In any case, the inquiry isn't generally why a few people are gay, however why our general public is hetero. Individuals naturally introduced to gay society, by and large, comply with the standard, similarly as do individuals naturally introduced to a hetero society. The vast majority of us have an expansive enough sexual reaction to enable us to be adapted serenely to either method of conduct. The individuals who feel less good with the norm, and the individuals who feel positive distress with it are not the slightest bit unnatural; rather, the limitations society puts on them that ought to be considered against nature.

One man in three has had some gay experience bringing about the climax, as per the Kinsey Report, distributed in 1948. Kinsey was not saying that one man in three was gay; however, he was removing the mark that marked sexuality between men as 'anomalous.' Kinsey called attention to that people were not the only ones among creatures in taking part in same-sex action: the supposition that creatures engaged in sexual relations just when proliferation could be ensured a human-made one, intended to support the view that homosexuality was 'against nature.' Fifty years have slipped by since the production of the Kinsey Report and socially acceptable sexual behaviors have changed. Be that as it may, Kinsey's discoveries still speak to an incredibly significant investigation into this zone of sexual conduct and the hidden patterns are as yet applicable today.

Gay experiences between men, for the most part, start in foreplay and end in the climax. Yet, the example of lovemaking is significantly less inflexible than the example of lovemaking among people will in general, be, and the two accomplices quite often arrive at the climax. Numerous gay men believe sex with other men to free because there are no standards: it doesn't include strain to perform or strain to fulfill the other individual and common fulfillment is easy because men see each other's bodies so well.

Men report that another bit of leeway of sex without commitments is that they believe they can come directly to the point; a sexual relationship frequently goes before a social fellowship, and not a different way. Numerous men depict their sexual relations with male accomplices as, for the most part, increasingly genuine and direct, both physically and inwardly than their associations with ladies.

Most gay men determine a lot of physical and passionate fulfillment from being infiltrated. Cleanliness ought to consistently be the primary need in any demonstration of butt-centric infiltration, as sickness is particularly. Effectively transmitted along these lines. Continuously wear a condom. A condom on a finger embedded into the butt can help grease just as a shield against scratches - from fingernails and unpleasant skin - that could prompt disease. You ought to consistently wash completely when butt-centric sex, and if you utilize a vibrator for entrance, ensure this is washed altogether as well, in hot lathery water with a sprinkle of germ-free included.

A few ladies oppose the thinness of business as usual and become lesbians for political reasons, feeling disappointed with a male overwhelmed society, others do so because they discover men inadmissible as darlings or as accomplices on an enthusiastic level, and others since they are seriously sincerely engaged with an individual from their very own sex and wish to express their sentiments through their sexuality.

CHAPTER NINE

KISSING

Kisses are cautiously organized overseen in the Kama Sutra. There's no going in all tongues blasting; you accumulate energy gradually: a brush of a lip here and a slip of the tongue there. Just certain pieces of the body ought to be kissed: brow, eyes, cheeks, throat, chest, bosoms, and the inside of the mouth.

There is an unbounded assortment of kisses that darlings can trade, from perky or delicate lip kissing to profoundly stirring open-mouth kissing with tongue play. Kissing somebody, you are distraught about is one of life's extraordinary delights - or ought to be. Shockingly enormous quantities of individuals have no clue how to kiss, and a poor kisser can be a horrendous disillusionment, similarly as somebody who is a gifted expert of the craft of kissing can make them detach your garments. The sweethearts' kiss or French kiss, including the entire mouth and tongue, is said to have its inceptions about how moms used to sustain their children in ancient societies. This training can be seen in laborer networks in certain pieces of Europe even today. The mother bites the nourishment for her infant before moving it legitimately from mouth to mouth she pushes her tongue, and the nourishment, inside the newborn child's mouth, and it responds with looking through developments of its tongue inside her mouth. Contemplations of cleanliness and the present relationship of mouth-to-mouth contact with sexual excitement make this nourishing unsuitable in our general public; however, the activity lives on in grown-up suggestive conduct.

A profound kiss is regularly the main shared affirmation that sexual fascination exists between a couple, and it is the primary component of sexuality to vanish from a relationship that is disappearing. As per Relate (the British Marriage Guidance Bureau), couples whose relationships are in a difficult situation are bound to have sex than to kiss. That mouth and tongue contact holds an uncommon closeness while intercourse can appear to be systematic, and the way likewise outlines remote that whores never kiss their customers.

The principal activity when kissing another darling is to discover with your lips and tongue where their teeth are, so you can abstain from hitting into them with your very own teeth. Conflicting teeth is as indifferent as conflicting display outlines. The following thing to recall is that kissing ought to be uncontrollably energizing: don't stall out stuck interminably rehashing a similar development, or your accomplice will lose focus and become exhausted. Shift the pace, and differ the activity, some of the time taking it, here and there being responsive to your accomplice.

Here are a couple of tips for progressively agreeable kissing:

- If your new accomplice doesn't smoke and you do, presently would be a generally excellent time to surrender the propensity. Non-smokers don't care for the taste or smell of tobacco.
- Until you must realize somebody well and they have guaranteed you they don't worry about it, don't eat solid tasting nourishment, for example, garlic or curry, except if your sweetheart is eating it as well.
- Oral cleanliness is significant. Ensure your mouth looks and tastes great. Get your dental specialist to de-scale your teeth consistently and eat a sound eating routine, so your breath is new.
- Do not kiss or have oral sex if you have a mouth or throat contamination. Kissing can move an expected 250 unique microbes and infections conveyed in spit; however, up 'til now, there is no proof to propose that AIDS can be trapped along these lines.
- Being kissed enthusiastically by a man with a stubble jawline isn't anyplace approach as sensual as being kissed energetically by a man who has as of late shaved.
- If you have facial hair, consider the way that it makes an obstruction between your skin and your lover's. There is no uncertainty that increasingly sensual contact is conceivable between a clean-shaven man and his accomplice.
- Women who wear make-up ought to be set up to have it licked off or, in any event, smeared. Think about how you feel about this before applying your make-up, yet whatever you do, don't leave yourself alone repressed by an impeccably painted face. Numerous men would like to kiss a face uncovered of make-up at any rate.
- To boost sensation when kissing, utilize every one of the muscles in your mouth and tongue. It is greatly improved kissing somebody whose mouth

reacts to yours and who realizes how to utilize pressure, then somebody whose mouth is fat and slack.

- Remember that nothing, however, nothing, is more regrettable than a slobbery kiss.

The ideal kiss

There are a couple of basic standards set down in the old writings to guarantee that each kiss motivates love as opposed to repugnance in your accomplice. A considerable lot of them remain constant today. The first is to ensure that you taste dazzling. The Kama Sutra prescribes eating betel leaves "together with different things that aroma the mouth." You should feel breath sure, nonetheless, with the contemporary identical: brushing, flossing, and mouthwash. The second is to utilize your teeth just as your lips and tongue. As per The Perfumed Garden, snacking a lady's lips creates a specific sort of salivation that is "sweet and perfect."

At long last, every one of the writings concurs that, if kissing makes you both woozy with want, you ought to line it up with sex, as The Perfumed Garden says: "Kisses are pointless if unaccompanied by the presentation of a penis... you ought to decline if you are not ready to have sexual intercourse or you will light a fire that solitary sterile partition can extinguish."

The kiss that dismisses

She kisses him delicately, however persistently when he's turning away from her. Her point is to dismiss his consideration from anything that he's doing, and spotlight everything on his or wants

The straight kiss

She squeezes her lips delicately against his as you both relish that first shiver of contact. Stroke each other with your breath as you scarcely contact one another. Keep the state of mind arousing and prodding: no tongues yet.

The incredibly squeezed kiss

In a snapshot of saucy closeness, he looks at her without flinching, moves back a bit, and squeezes her lower lip between his thumb and finger. He, at that point, follows up by squeezing his lips firmly against hers.

The catching kiss

She grasps his head and takes the two his lips between hers, sucking them and stroking them with her tongue. She, at that point, places her tongue in his mouth and twines it around his.

The kiss of the upper lip

He encases her upper lip among his, and she kisses his lower lip. Let the tip of your tongue tantalizingly brush your darling's lip (yet keep the tongue contacts light and intermittent).'

The twisted kiss

At long last, when the bait of a tongue-twining kiss gets powerful, he squeezes his lips against hers, and she points her head to the side. You close your eyes, part your lips, and put it all on the line.

CHAPTER TEN

PREMATURE EJACULATION

Nervousness is regularly the reason for untimely discharge. In an extramarital relationship, a man may discharge when he infiltrates his accomplice's vagina, in spite of the way that he doesn't have this issue with his significant other. This is an indication of blame. A man may likewise discharge before he wishes to on the off chance that he feels startled that his method isn't adequate, and discharging rapidly will keep him from uncovering his absence of experience.

Accepting that sex is terrible as a result of what you were told as a kid is another conceivable reason for untimely discharge. On the off chance that as a kid, you were rebuffed for stroking off, you may have trained yourself to come rapidly to reduce the opportunity of being discovered and to limit the blame you felt at your very own pleasure.

The dread of getting excessively near someone else may likewise be a contributing variable. Closeness consistently carries with it the danger of misfortune, and the excruciating agony orderly on that misfortune. Intuitively, a man who gets sex over with rapidly might be attempting to shield himself from a close enthusiastic association.

A few procedures can assist men with enduring longer, and these ought to be utilized related to analyzing the reason for the issue. Understanding what's up regularly brings its very own discharge.

The stop-start procedure for postponing the discharge
The point of these activities is to figure out how to keep yourself beneath the time when discharge appears to be unavoidable for whatever length of time that conceivable. Men who don't have an accomplice can rehearse the initial three stages. In themselves, they will assist you with increasing a more prominent proportion of control. For the last four stages, you will require the co-activity of an accomplice.

Stage one

Jerk off with a dry hand. Abstain from fantasizing, and focus rather on the sensation in your penis. Enable the joy to develop yet stop promptly; you believe you are going to lose control. Unwind for some time, as yet keeping your mind free of dreams, until the threat of discharge has passed, at that point start once more, following a similar example, plan to keep halting and beginning for 15 minutes without climax. You will be unable to oversee it from the start, yet continue attempting. As you get increasingly rehearsed, you will most likely discover you need to stop less frequently. At the point when you have finished three 15-minute sessions on three continuous events (not one following the other!), continue to stage two.

Stage two

Includes jerking off with a greasing up jam to elevate sensation, and make postpone progressively troublesome. Pursue the system in stage one until you have finished three separate continuous sessions as above.

Stage three

You will currently have increased a decent proportion of control. The following stage includes stroking off with a dry hand for 15 minutes before discharge. Continue concentrating on your penis as opposed to fantasizing. At the point when you feel yourself getting hazardously energized, don't stop, yet rather, change musicality or adjust your strokes so that the strain to discharge blurs. Examination to see which strokes energize you most, and which permit you the most control. Work on this progression until you have finished three successive sessions as in the past.

Stage four

Presently include your accomplice. Lie on your back and get her to jerk off you with a dry hand, as in stage one. Focus on the sensations in your penis and request that she stop each time you get excessively excited before the 15 minutes is up. The point is to keep going for three continuous 15-minute sessions.

Stage five

Rehash stage four, however, request that your accomplice utilize an oil while she jerks off you. You will discover discharge considerably more hard to control, and you may need to request that she stop all the more regularly. When you have aced three successive 15-minute sessions, you are prepared to attempt the stop-start system with intercourse.

Stage Six

The best position for deferring discharge is with the lady on top. When you are inside her, request that her move tenderly. Put your hands on her hips so you can tell her with your hands when you need her to stop, and when you are prepared for her to begin once more. Once more, expect to keep going for 15 minutes, yet on the off chance that you can't, don't stress; you can begin again once you recuperate your erection, and the second time you will likely have more control. During intercourse, focus altogether on yourself. Give your accomplice your full fixation and carry her to climax either previously or a short time later, with oral or manual incitement.

Stage seven

Proceed onward to different positions. It is progressively hard to delay - discharge with the man on top, so spare this until last.

The press strategy for deferring discharge

The 'press' activity is intended to make your erection die down, and it tends to be applied each time you get excessively near discharge. Your accomplice plays out the crush by holding your penis solidly and squeezing with her thumb on the frenulum. This is the spot on the underside of the penis where the head joins the pole. Simultaneously, she pushes on the contrary side of the penis with her pointer, and with her different fingers twisted around the pole. It is significant that she presses genuinely hard on the penis and doesn't move her hand at the same time.

Too light a touch could make you discharge straight away.

Stage one

Get your accomplice to jerk off you with a dry hand. Whenever you get excessively near discharge, sign to her to stop and crush your penis. Similarly, as with the stop-start procedure, we intend to keep going for three back to back 15minute sessions before proceeding onward to stage two.

Stage two

Get your accomplice to jerk off you gradually and tenderly as in the past, yet this time requests that her utilization an ointment. Pursue the technique for stage one.

Stage three

Presently you are prepared for intercourse, however not for pushing, rather, lie on your back and request that your accomplice sits over you, with your penis inside her. Neither of you should move. When you want to come, your accomplice should ascend off you (this development is risky as it applies incitement), and quickly hold your penis in the crushing grasp. Rehash the activity two or multiple times before you enable yourself to discharge.

Stage four

At the point when you feel progressively certain about your poise, request that your accomplice move delicately while she sits over you similarly situated. At the point when you want to discharge, she should get off you and press as in the past, until you can most recent 15 minutes without discharging.

Stage five

You are currently prepared to attempt different positions, yet recall that with the man on top, you will have the least control. Similarly, as with the stop-start system, during intercourse, you should concentrate on yourself. Your accomplice won't feel dismissed on the off chance that you carry her to climax orally or physically either previously or after intercourse.

Thinking about Birth Control

Considering anti-conception medication is a piece of contemplating engaging in sexual relations. A few people decide to connect just in sexual practices other than intercourse - some since they favour different types of closeness; some since they're not prepared for intercourse; and some since they would prefer not to chance pregnancy.

Picking a strategy for anti-conception medication isn't, in every case simple. Notwithstanding pondering the adequacy, advantages, and conceivable symptoms of the techniques you're thinking about, you have to consider what you feel good utilizing. It's essential to ask yourself what strategies practically fit with your character and way of life. Discussing conception prevention with an accomplice can be hard. It might attempt to sift through your very own emotions before you raise the subject with your accomplice. Attempt to discover a period and an approach to discuss it that feels good to you.

What Do Effectiveness Rates Mean?

A scope of viability is recorded for every technique for conception prevention in this present. The lower rating recorded is the "run of the mill viability," which considers inaccurate or conflicting use. The higher number is the "hypothetical adequacy" rate, which depicts the technique's viability when utilized accurately every time a few engages in sexual relations. Adequacy measurements are hard to assess because they change generally relying upon the structure of the exploration study. The strategy with the most elevated adequacy rating might be the "best" technique for you. The best technique is the one which you are educated about, OK with, and will utilize reliably.

Conception prevention and Sexually Transmitted Diseases (STDs)

You might be fundamentally worried about forestalling pregnancy when you pick a strategy for anti-conception medication. Yet, on the off chance that you or your accomplice has ever had sexual contact with any other person, you might be in danger of getting an STD. Utilizing condoms and spermicide gives the best assurance against STDs. Different techniques for conception prevention (noted in this present) may likewise give some assurance. Numerous ladies and men use condoms and spermicide alongside different strategies for anti-conception medication to shield themselves and their accomplices from STDs.

Imagine a scenario in which Your Method Fails.

Right and reliable utilization of your contraception technique makes it more averse to come up short, be that as it may, no strategy is great. On the off chance that your strategy comes up short or you have unprotected intercourse, the danger of pregnancy might be decreased by quickly embeddings two uses of spermicide into the vagina. Likewise, call the Gynecology Clinic or Dial-A-Nurse about the accessibility of a next day contraceptive.

Sex helps and aphrodisiacs

An assortment of sex helps or toys are sold over-the-counter in sex shops or via mail requests through magazines. These incorporate Chinese balls (a lady can wear them in her vagina where they vibrate somewhat as she moves about during the day) and condoms with different distensions on them, which are intended to invigorate the clitoris during intercourse. Different condoms are brilliantly shaded and seasoned with organic products.

The vibrator is, by a long shot, the most well-known sex toy. Molded as a penis and battery-ope evaluated, it tends to be utilized in adoration play or for female masturbation. A few vibrators have a discharge component. Many sex specialists educate the utilization regarding a vibrator for ladies figuring out how to give themselves climaxes.

To help look after erection, the straightforward ring intended to fit at the base of the penis is likely the main valuable gadget. A bit of strip will do similarly well. Tied reasonably firmly around the penis, it goes about as a single direction valve. Blood enters the penis yet is kept from leaving it, and hence the erection is kept up for somewhat more. An assortment of creams and showers that guarantee to drag out erections or to trigger climaxes are likewise accessible.

Named after Aphrodite, the Greek goddess of affection, aphrodisiacs are drugs professed to energize desire. They may likewise be taken to fight off depletion or uplift delight during sex. The fame of these medications since the beginning is a declaration to the whimsicalness of human sexual science.

In certain civic establishments, exceptionally nutritious nourishments were viewed as the most dependable energizers, and may to be sure, have beneficially affected individuals whose diet was typically poor. The Greeks went for eggs, nectar, snails, and shellfish, for example, mussels and crabs. One Arab formula from The Perfumed Garden suggests a glass of exceptionally thick nectar, twenty almonds and a hundred pine nuts be taken for three evenings on resigning. Different plans were to be applied remotely. To build the elements of little individuals and make them unbelievable', the creator of The Perfumed Garden prompted scouring the penis with the dissolved down fat from the mound of a camel, wounded bloodsuckers, asses' individuals, and even hot pitch. These 'rubs' were most likely less powerful than the treatment of scouring itself.

The Chinese were progressively logical in their methodology. They estimated and mixed the powdered underlying foundations of plants; at that point gave them beautiful names like 'the uncovered chicken medication.' This medication got its name when a septuagenarian government worker who took it routinely, fathered three children and gave such a great amount of consideration to his significant other that she could never again either sit or rests. He had to toss the remaining parts of the medication out into the yard, where it was eaten up by the cockerel. The rooster hopped on a hen straight away and kept mating with it for a few days without interference, at the same time pecking at its head to keep its equalization, until the chicken was uncovered, at which point the cockerel tumbled off. The glad creator of the medication guaranteed that on the off chance that it was taken three times each day for sixty days, a man would have the option to fulfill 40 ladies.

Horns have, for quite some time, been thought to have Spanish fly properties in light of their conspicuous phallic shape. Proceeding with confidence in the intensity of rhinoceros horn has brought the single-horned African rhinoceros to the verge of elimination. Horn comprises of sinewy tissue, comparable in development to hair and nails. Like them, rhino horn contains the protein keratin, and the minerals sulfur, calcium, and phosphorus. The expansion of these components to a less than stellar eating routine may improve life, yet a cheddar sandwich would do similarly too.

Another well-known love potion is Spanish fly, the regular name of the creepy-crawly cantharides. The creepy crawly is dried, and the dynamic head, cantharidin, is removed. Whenever gulped, cantharidin creates an extreme consuming uproar in the throat, trailed by the runs. At that point, the urinogenital tract turns out to be aroused to such an extent that pee gets inconceivable. The penis winds up engorged and throbbing, yet this is because of horrifying torment as opposed to sexual earnestness. Taking Spanish fly can, at times, be lethal.

Explicitly transmitted ailments

The SYMPTOMS of sexually transmitted diseases (STD) are frequently difficult to distinguish at first, however in the event that your accomplice is contaminated, or you have a sexual association with somebody who is indiscriminate; at that point registration is basic. In the event that side effects do show themselves, they are probably going to appear as a release from the vagina, penis or rear-end, or tingling or irritation around the private parts or rear-end, or irregularity or rash on the privates, butt or mouth.

Continuously utilize a condom. If you speculate you may have an explicitly transmitted ailment, you should see your primary care physician or center straight away. You can discover the phone number of your closest center by looking into 'unique facility,' 'venereal sickness' or 'VD' in the phone catalogue, or by calling your nearby clinic. You will be tried as fast as could reasonably be expected, and if the test is certain, you will be encouraged to contact your ongoing sexual accomplices, as they also may require treatment. Maintain a strategic distance from sex until you are clear of the sickness.

Continuously utilize a condom. AIDS represents Acquired Immune Deficiency Syndrome, and the malady is brought about by the human immuno-inadequacy infection, known as HIV Once it is inside the body, this infection attacks the white platelets, which ordinarily fend off illness; at that point, it increases and crushes them. It likewise breeds inside the mind. Three to four years regularly slip by between contamination with HIV and any ensuing improvement of the indications related to AIDS.

As AIDS builds up the body's regular guards, become drained, and the AIDS quiet is progressively liable to contract ailments that a sound body would ordinarily avoid, thus uncommon types of malignant growth and pneumonia create. Once in awhile AIDS patients are assaulted by a few diseases on the double, for example, candida, herpes, and TB. Simultaneously, the mind may capitulate to progressively serious dementia. Somewhere close to one out of ten and one out of three of those contaminated with HIV are probably going to create AIDS. So far, there is no solution to AIDS. It helps, as a rule, advances through different contaminations and phases of expanding debility to the possible passing of the sufferer.

Instructions to stay away from AIDS

- Always utilize a condom
- Avoid butt-centric sex
- Always utilize a condom
- Don't share toothbrushes, razors, or whatever other instruments that may move blood from cuts or scraped spots.

The infection is available in body liquids, essentially semen, and blood. It might likewise be available in spit, however, inquire about demonstrates that salivation appears to show little hazard. Having butt-centric intercourse with a contaminated accomplice is the doubtless method for getting AIDS, and 80 percent of British cases so far have been male gay people.

The second most normal method for getting the malady is through contaminated blood. Just about a fourth of Britain's hemophiliac populaces presently convey HIV since they have been infused with the coagulating specialist gathered from tainted blood. (Hemophiliacs are conceived without the blood-coagulating factor and can experience the ill effects of minor damage, and seep to death from a cut except if they get the thickening variable from giving blood.) HIV in the blood may likewise be transmitted on tainted needles, and medication addicts are the third most profoundly in danger gathering of the populace.

To become HIV positive, you don't need to be gay or unbridled, a medication fanatic or a hemophiliac. Heteros are likewise in danger. Indeed, even a hetero in an unfaltering relationship stands the danger of getting the illness if their accomplice has been tainted in a past relationship. Hence while leaving on any new relationship, it is most secure to wear a condom.

Gonorrhea is brought about by the bacterium gonococcus, which can't get by outside the body and is transmitted uniquely by sex, and never (as is now and then envisioned) on latrine seats or towels. In men, the urethra, along which pee goes from the bladder, is tainted, and there is here and there torment on peeing and a thick release from the penis inside seven days after disease. In gay men, the rectum might be contaminated, with the probability of disturbance and release from the butt. In ladies, gonorrhea taints the cervix, urethra, and rectum, and, similarly, as with men, there might be release and agony on peeing. On the off chance that disease spreads to the uterus, there is a 10 percent chance that the fallopian cylinders might be blocked, causing sterility. Regularly, be that as it may, there are no manifestations in either men or ladies.

The treatment for gonorrhea is typically a solitary portion of anti-infection agents, for example, penicillin, with a registration a while later to ensure the contamination has cleared. If gonorrhea isn't analyzed and treated, genuine intricacies can create. Men may endure epicliclymitis - agony and grow in the balls; ladies may endure peritonitis - irritation of the films of the stomach area. Both genders could create gonococcal septicemia, contamination of the circulatory system with skin rashes, and joint inflammation. In genuine cases, sterility can bring about both genders. Pregnant ladies with gonorrhea may give it to their children, who can be brought into the world with gonococcal ophthalmia, an intense irritation of the eyes. Complexities are, notwithstanding, generally uncommon these days.

Vague urethritis or NSU can be recognized by bumps, irritation, or tingling around the privates, rear-end, or mouth. There may likewise be a release from the vagina or penis. The treatment is generally a fourteen-day course of anti-microbials for any individual who has had contact with a contaminated individual. During treatment, patients 0are approached to surrender liquor, as this can achieve a repeat of the manifestations. Intricacies can happen, and these are like those for gonorrhea, yet luckily early determination and treatment can avert these. It is workable for a man to be occasionally reinfected with NSU without changing his sex accomplice, and no clarification has so far been advanced for this. Be that as it may, the two accomplices will require treatment each time NSU shows itself.

Syphilis is very uncommon in Britain today. It influences ladies not as much as men, and its fundamental unfortunate casualties are male gay people. Indications show up between 10 days and 12 weeks after disease. In the essential phase of the sickness, a little hard sore or chancre shows up on the penis, vagina, or rectum. It is effortless and ordinarily vanishes rapidly. Half a month later, in the auxiliary stage, the patient is hot, with swollen organs and tingling skin. The ailment is reparable with anti-infection agents, however in the event that for reasons unknown it ought not to be dealt with, genuine difficulties will create numerous years after the fact. Until the approach of anti-toxins, tertiary syphilis used to be very normal, with patients, in the long run, experiencing dementia and dying in some horrible, nightmarish way a moderate, anguishing demise.

Chlamycliais one of the most well-known STDs and is brought about by a bacterial parasite called chlamydia trachomatis. The sickness is analyzed by a swab test, and treatment is with anti-infection agents. Side effects in men incorporate a whitish-yellow release from the penis, visit 'consuming' pee, and redness at the tip of the penis. Ladies may see a release, a regular need to pee, and gentle uneasiness which they may confuse with vaginitis or menstrual spasms. However, many ladies experience no side effects until they create inconveniences, for example, pelvic fiery sickness, a genuine condition that can bring about barrenness. Infants destined to tainted moms may experience the ill effects of eye contamination, which is in some cases genuine, or pneumonia.

Genital herpes is a viral contamination transmitted through sex. It is fundamentally the same as the other kind of herpes, which causes mouth blisters, and can likewise be gotten by having oral sex with somebody who has dynamic mouth blisters. The side effects are tingling, torment in the crotch, uneasiness on peeing and fever, trailed by the presence of excruciating red rankles on the vulva or penis, which burst to frame ulcers. After around 10 days the manifestations vanish and the patient seems, by all accounts, to be relieved. In any case, the contamination is just lying lethargic and may repeat whenever, especially when the patient is under pressure. There is so far no treatment for this ailment. While the ailment is torpid, it is sheltered to engage in sexual relations without contaminating one's accomplice, however, it is difficult to anticipate the following assault, so the danger of disease remains. On the off chance that the disease is dynamic toward the finish of a pregnancy, a Cesarean area might be performed to avoid the infant getting tainted in the birth channel.

Genital moles are unsavory however easy and can be dealt with effectively. They are little irregularities that show up on the penis, vulva, or butt and are somewhat infectious. The treatment includes either painting the moles with planning called podophyllin or solidifying them off with fluid nitrogen. The affiliation has been recognized between genital moles and cervical malignant growth, so it is critical to dispose of them at the earliest opportunity and to have normal cervical smears.

Thrush is a contagious disease that creates specific conditions in the vagina. It is here and there connected to taking the Pill, and in the event that it repeats often, an alternate technique for contraception might be fitting. A man may convey thrush, however, he typically shows no indications. Thrush causes vaginal irritation and tingling, and a thick white release. The specialist will most likely endorse hostile to contagious cream, to be utilized by the two accomplices, and vaginal pessaries, however, oral medicines are accessible as well. A few ladies locate that characteristic yogurt in the vagina is successful. Dodge hot showers, and wearing tights, tight pants, and nylon pants.

Trichomoniasis is one of the most widely recognized and least genuine of all explicitly transmitted ailments and might be passed on by terrible cleanliness practice in the utilization of towels just as by sexual contact. It can exist in a symptom-free frame and a few people go about as inactive bearers for the ailment. Be that as it may, it can likewise cause release and agony in peeing in both genders. A few medications are accessible for treatment and their prosperity rate is high.

Back rub strokes

Stroking and scouring were indispensable pre-sex warm-ups in the East. Ladies, particularly, were believed to need a man's strokes and touches to get them in the temperament. Attempt a couple of these back rub procedures to demonstrate that men are similarly as defenseless to alluring strokes as ladies.

Liquefying knead

Make your pre-sex knead sexy instead of clinical with heaps of warm scented oil. Empty some into your hands, rub them together, and afterward let your palms skim easily over your sweetheart's skin. Or then again delicately warm the oil on a radiator, and sprinkle it straight on. Commit whole back rub sessions to their pleasure. Unadulterated joy implies having the option to unwind in the information that you won't need to get up in a moment and give back in kind. Also, be inventive. Your hands are only one back rub apparatus available to you. Others incorporate your hair, your fingernails, your feet, even your breath. Make your darling shudder and shiver with delight.

Single-word of caution: don't press on joints or bones, or your accomplice is bound to jump than soften. On the off chance that you rub your sweetheart's back, touch the muscles on either side of the spine, yet abstain from squeezing the spine straightforwardly.

Turning up the warmth

Increment the suggestion of your back rub as you sense your darling getting progressively loose and malleable. For instance, as you stroke the tummy, you can let your hand brush nearer and nearer to their private parts. Or on the other hand, you can improve a leg knead with some scarcely there kisses on the inward thighs.

Scalp orbiting

She presses the stack of her fingers against his sanctuaries and moves them in moderate, firm circles. She moves her fingers all over his scalp, hovering as she goes, just as tenderly washing his hair.

Shoulder rub

He squeezes his thumbs into the muscles at the rear of her shoulder and his fingers into the plunge simply over her collarbone. He at that point works for his hands in moderate, roundabout manipulating developments.

Bosom strokes

Keeping his hands level, he slides his palms over her body and over the bends of her bosoms; he utilizes his thumb and forefinger in a scissor activity over her areolas, pressing delicately as he goes.

Bum manipulating

She inclines forward with the goal that her chest area weight is on her hands. She at that point plies and presses his muscles utilizing the tips of her fingers, the impact points of her hands, and the level piece of her clench hands.

Calf pressure

She chips away at his huge lower leg muscles by sliding her fingers here and there in contradicting bearings, orbiting her thumbs, and rounding her fingertips crosswise over up ripping at the movement.

Foot-warmers

He gives her an agreeable foot press with his thumbs on her underside and his fingers on the highest point of her foot. He at that point floats his thumbs along the base of her foot and squeezes and presses every one of her toes.

CHAPTER ELEVEN

UNDRESSING EACH OTHER

In the Kama Sutra, each sexual demonstration from kissing to scratching is performed with cautious and respectful service, and uncovering is no special case. So in case, you're prone to rip off one another's garments in a sex-hungry furor, follow some guidelines from Vatsyayana's experience: transform uncovering into a suggestive ceremony.

Stripped joy

Rather than review taking each other's garments off as the exhausting however important piece, treat it as a major aspect of foreplay. Envision you're taking the wrapping off the hottest blessing wrapped present ever. Each time you uncover another piece of your sweetheart's body, feast upon it with your lips, tongue, teeth, hands, and eyes. As you smooth her legging down her thigh or his jeans over his hips, abuse the chance to brush nearby problem areas with your fingertips. Slow things down, and reveal each piece of your darling's body with a feeling of amazement.

Tips for being stripped

Focus on the unobtrusive yet heavenly impression of your garments being stripped or pulled away from your skin. On the off chance that your sweetheart stalls out on a catch or affixing, don't attempt to help; give up to their control. Wear hot or exotic textures that your sweetheart will take pleasure in contacting: for instance, silk, trim, cowhide, or latex. Furthermore, grasp the sensual intensity of flashes by wearing thigh-high hurdle up boots; dresses with zips that run from the neck to fix; or zippable undergarments, catsuits, basques, or pockets (for him).

Uncovering her: Off the shoulder He gives her goose pimples as he nestles and licks the rear of her neck, simultaneously, he slides her dress off her shoulder to uncover its smooth bend

Uncovering him: Baring his chest she fixes his shirt catches with hot gradualness, inclining in to touch his chest with her lips after each catch, lighting his fire and making him consider what might be on the horizon.

Stripping her: Slow disclosing! Having fixed her bra, he cups her bosoms through the texture, daintily scanning for her areolas with his fingertips, at that point tweaking and squeezing them. He at that point slides the bra down over her shoulders

Uncovering her: Reveal all He stoops compliantly at her feet before taking the texture of her undies between his teeth, he at that point edges her undies gradually down her thighs; far and away superior if she is wearing drawstring clothing.

Uncovering him: On the fly, she looks brazenly up at him from a stooping situation as she fixes his flies and facilitates his pants over his abdomen, her lips tantalizingly near his groin

Disrobing him: Grand finale She slides her hands provocatively under the edge of his jeans for a brisk bum touch, at that point with an energetic grin she smoothest his jeans gradually over his hips

Gnawing, scratching, and striking

As indicated by the Kama Sutra, denoting your darling with teeth and nails is an indication of serious energy. In the event that your accomplice is probably going to be disturbed or annoyed instead of stimulated, don't think about this stuff. However, in case you're both into it, the "blows of affection" can make hot increments to your enticement collection.

Making your imprint

Test-drive your sweetheart's energy by consolidating the odd hit or scratch into a back rub or sex. Attempt a few nips, hits, or scratches in places where they can be concealed by garments. An openly noticeable love nibble may send your darling shouting, in any case, as the Kama Sutra says, seeing blemishes on shrouded places brings back recollections of adoration and enthusiasm.

Keeping it fun-loving

No nonsense sex is a certain something; awakening beat up is another. A few people wear nibbles, scratches, and other sex wounds with sensual pride; others flinch with shame. Check which bunch your darling falls into before letting tear.

Take off rings and wrist trinkets before a beating session. What's more, discover how hard your sweetheart likes their base hit on a 1–5 scale: "1" is a delicate love pat and "5" is a whack that stings and leaves you to read in the two arrangements of cheeks. You should ignore the Kama Sutra proposal of cutting the nails of your left hand into focuses (except if you're into serious agony during nail play). Rather, simply pursue your mum's recommendation, and keep your nails perfect and cut into delicate bends.

The gnawing of a hog

He energetically nibbles her shoulder and along her arm, abandoning a progression of dark red imprints. The Kama Sutra prescribes this for "people of extreme enthusiasm".

Half-moon

She squeezes her nails into his rear end and leaves half-moon shapes engraved on his tissue. (The Kama Sutra additionally prescribes making circles: two half-moons inverse one another.)

Broken cloud

He squeezes his mouth to her skin (anyplace on her body), sucks her tissue tenderly, at that point chomps and snack to desert an imprint looking like a broken cloud.

Strike

She pretends outrage and strikes him on the chest with the rear of her hand (she can join this into pretend situations). On the off chance that he prefers it, she rehashes it while getting increasingly "furious"

Forehand strike

He marginally cups his hand and slaps her energetically on the bum at short proximity. He at that point lines it up with a calming butt cheek rub, before giving a beat to the next cheek.

CONCLUSION

In conclusion, no single position is more moral or normal than another is. If you truly enjoy one position, that's great. If not, then try something else or something unique. Thanks so much for your time!!!

Printed in Great Britain
by Amazon